Self-healing Guide

. . . for beginners . . .

Dr. Shiv Dua

HEALTH ❧ HARMONY

An imprint of

B. Jain Publishers (P) Ltd.

An ISO 9001 : 2000 Certified Company

USA — EUROPE — INDIA

Note from the Publishers

Any information given in this book is not intended to be taken as a replacement for medical advice. Any person with condition requiring medical attention should consult a qualified practitioner or therapeutist.

Homoeopathic
SELF-HEALING GUIDE
for beginners

Reprint Edition: 2007
First Edition: 2005

Published by **Kuldeep Jain** *for*

HEALTH 🌳 HARMONY

an imprint of **B. Jain Publishers (P) Ltd.**
1921, Street No. 10, Chuna Mandi,
Paharganj, New Delhi–110 055 (INDIA)
Phones: 91-011-2358 0800, 2358 1100, 2358 1300
Fax: 91-011-2358 0471; Email: bjain@vsnl.com
Website: www.bjainbooks.com

Printed in India by
J. J. Offset Printers
522, FIE, Patpar Ganj, Delhi–110 092
Phones: 91-011-2216 9633, 2215 6128

BOOK CODE / ISBN: 978-81-319-0228-8

The book especially suits to people . . .

- Who desire to learn Homoeopathy for self-treatment.
- Who care for their health and the health of their family-members as well.
- Who wish to cure disorders and acute diseases at home.
- Who are BHMS students, learning homoeopathy in college.
- Who have finished BHMS and are going to start their own practice.

Emergencies :
When to Rush to a Qualified Homoeopath . . .

* The patient appears to be very sick and his/ her symptoms are not easily understood.

* The nature of disease is not understood.

* There is profuse bleeding (unexplained), from any part of the body or skin.

* The patient is restless; his/her breathing is rapid, shallow or too slow.

* The diarrhoea is of long standing nature, along with severe weakness.

* Delirium or convulsions exist.

* Pain in stomach or abdomen is too severe, persistent and there is no relief after 15-20 minutes of giving medicine to the patient.

* Continuous vomiting and vertigo exist.

* Vomiting starts after the onset of viral disease.

* Chest pain is severe and extending to arms, back and shoulders.

* The patient becomes senseless.

* The temperature is high above104°F and pulse is slow.

* Fever is lasting for more than five days.

* There is continuous low fever for more than 15 days.

* Headache is so severe that the patient cries like a child.

* The patient is very much confused and upset mentally and he/she is not able to describe his/her symptoms.

* Urine is pale, dark or having blood in it.

- Urine is profuse and is uncontrollable
- Urine is scanty, with pain; or there is retention of urine for more than two hours.
- Extreme weakness to the extent of falling exists.
- Cough with wheezing exists for more than 10 days.
- Skin or white part of eyes become yellow.
- Body becomes rigid or neck is stiff for more than two hours.
- Stools are yellow and having streak or flow of blood.
- There are lumps, cysts, growths, long standing warts and moles or the case is of deep- seated skin disease or long standing ulcers of stomach.
- The disease is chronic and of long standing nature.

About the author . . .

DR. SHIV DUA, M.A., D.I.Hom. HMD (London) is a well-known name in the literacy circles of Homoepathy. His four books, 'Practitioners Guide to Gall bladder and Kidney Stone', 'Oral Diseases', 'Cervical Spondylosis-Neck Pain' and 'Know and Solve Thyroid Problems' have been published. To his credit are more than hundred Hindi articles on homoeopathy that were published in leading Rajasthan newspapers like 'Rajasthan Patrika' and 'Denik Bhasker'. Homoeopathic Sandesh, a mouth organ of Delhi Homoeopathic Medical association published more than fifty articles in Hindi and English. His contribution of homoeopathic articles to magazines like 'Homoeopathic Heritage', 'Vital Informer' and 'Homoeopathy for All' is a continuous flow from time to time. His articles printed in souvenirs of various seminars carry weight. He has been delivering lectures on various subjects on Homoeopathy in scientific meetings of HMAI, Faridabad, HMAI, Aligarh, DHMA, New Delhi and in the recent past and an active participant in seminars and meetings for the benefit of the profession. He is Secretary (Literacy), HMAI, Faridabad, Haryana unit and member of DHMA and SDHA New Delhi. At present he is Homoeopathic Medical Officer at Arya Samaj charitable Hospital, Sector 19, Faridabad.

Dedicated To . . .

THIS BOOK is dedicated to my respected father and teacher in homoeopathy, Late Shri Hira Nand Dua. He taught me my first and last lesson in life, work hard and still work hard. We were the victims of Indo-Pak partition and faced poverty boldly. I was the only son of my parents and was seven years old when partition took place. Unaware of hardships of life, I had a glorious rich childhood in Pakistan as my father ran a roaring dry fruit business in oil Mandi, Bannu, NWFP. He was matriculate, which was considered good qualification during those days. In India, we landed at Amritsar and my father got a job of accountant (eighty rupees a month) at a publisher's shop. Besides accounting, he read proofs, translated and wrote storybooks for children. His Hindi-English translator (Publishers- M/s Prem Singh Sachdev and sons, *Bazar Mai Sewan*, Amritsar) was a popular book of the times. To help run the household expenses, my mother, four sisters and I did all types of jobs at home including folding and sewing printed papers, binding books, make fancy items (like 'Rakhi') and paper- envelops. During vacations, I worked as a hawker in the streets of Amritsar to sell mill-cloth, which I used to carry on my head and shoulders. Expenses on study in school and college for all the children were partly borne by my father, my elder sister and myself by coaching tuitions to lower class students. When I did my matriculation, I learnt typing and started part time work as typist with one lawyer and also as desk-accountant at a firm dealing in supply of straw boards. Important of all was our homoeopathy. Inspite of the fact that my father was short of funds, he stored homoeopathic, unani and biochemic medicines to practice on charitable basis at home. Initially, our patients were neighbours, the families living in our street and then the labourers working in bookshops of *Bazar Mai Sewan*. Those days, that *Bazar* was full of bookshops only. Great Gurumukhi writer Nanak Singh had a bookshop there.

It was my duty to make doses of pills and powders in folded papers and tell patients how to take the medicines. My father had many 'Urdu' books on homoeopathic and Unani system of medicines. He used to bring variety of books at home for our reading. My sisters and I read almost all classic writers like Rabinder Nath Tagore, Sharat Chand, Bankim Chander, and Prem chand, Gorkey, Dostoevesky and others. Magical novels (Tilasami) like Bhoot nath and Chanderkanta running into tens of volumes were our favourite. I was so much fascinated by the world of books that I started writing poems and stories. My first Hindi story, 'Prayshchit' was published in daily 'Hindi Milap' when I was twelve years old. The very first medicine book that fascinated me was an Urdu book 'Asli Kamil Sanyasi' in which hundreds of domestic and unani medicines were given for all ailments. The book written by Hakim Diwan Kahan chand Kapoor of Lahore was published in December 1924 and I still have it in my library. The pictures of various organs of human body are roughly pen-sketched in the beginning of book and my childlike curiousity found those sketches fascinating. The formulae (*nuskhe*) given in the book are very useful. I still remember taking grounded powder of *'Pipal' tree-leaf and skin of tree with honey for stomatitis.* This formula given on page 165 of the book is very effective for children who suffer from frequent *mouth ulcers.*

My father was a writer, homoeopath, scholar, competent wrestler, swimmer and very pious man attending both Arya Samaj and Gurudwara Golden temple regularly. He knew five languages, Hindi, Urdu, Gurumukhi, English and Pashto (language of Afganistan). He struggled hard and amidst adversity, he never lost his patience to rebuild a second coming in India. He used to say that:

"No work is mean or degraded even if we work as labourers."

I joined as a labourer in Indian Bureau of Mines on daily wages at the rate of Rupees two per day for learning drilling work on machines (mineral investigations). Living away from home in jungles of Rajasthan, my technical and academic studies continued in tents burning real mid night oil. In course of time, I was regularized as a drilling assistant and then promoted to Jr. Tech. Assistant. I left I.B.M. and joined Geological Survey of India, Calcutta as a Driller (Class II gazetted post). During my service time itself; I did Honours in Hindi, M.A in English and D.I.Hom. and D.H.M. (British Institute of Homoeopathy, London through M/s B. Jain Publishers). I had plenty of time in jungles and villages to devote to the cause of homoeopathy. Medical facilities for poor villagers in the remote jungles did not exist and this gave me opportunity to treat them through homoeopathic medicines.

My father was always in touch with me through his inspiring letters, insisting me to study whenever I faced failures in treatment of patients. In one of his letters, he wrote, "Persons, who have passion for work, should always put in their best efforts and senses in the job at hand. Success cannot be far away".

Dr. Shiv Dua
M.A., D.I.Hom., D.H.M. (London)
RHMP: B-4048 (Haryana)

Gratitude . . .

* I am thankful to Mr. Kuldeep Jain for his continued encouragement in writing this little work on homoeopathy. A towering publishing house like B.Jain Publishers has been like a blessing to Homoeopathy in enlarging its image and a boon for writers who want to expose their skills. M/s B.Jain Publishers have already published my four books, 'Gall Bladder and Kidney Stones', 'Oral Diseases', 'Cervical Spondylosis' and 'Know and Solve Thyroid Problems'. I am obliged to the readers and thank them for the interest they have shown in my first book on gall bladder and kidney stones, which is now in its second edition.

* I shall be failing in my duty if I do not thank the members of my family, Uma, Dharmesh, Anu, Akshay and Aryan whose help enabled me to work on writing job.

* I am also thankful to Mr. and Mrs. H.K. Rawal, Amit, Nilima and Tanya for their whole heartly support in achieving this writing.

* My sincere thanks to Major K.C. Virmani, Mrs. Raj Virmani and family for keen interest in my books and homoeopathy. Mrs. Raj Virmani is a good homoeopath also.

* I am thankful to Mr. Gyan Budhiraja, Indu, Deepak, Sangeeta, Pardeep and Charu for their help and encouragement for writing this book.

* I shall also not be out of way to thank Dr. Sanjeev Kumar, BHMS, gold medalist, Faridabad for the help he has been rendering from time to time through meaningful discussions and suggestions on various subjects relating to homoeopathic medicines.

* It is my duty to thank Dr. D.K. Mukherjee, Jaipur/Kolkata for his kind help and association in treating hundreds of patients during year 1995-1997 at Kalibari Homoeopathic Charitable Hospital, Kali Mandir, Malviya Nagar, Jaipur.

* My sincere thanks to Dr. Mukesh Mathur, the then Medical officer, Rukmadevi Bajaj Dharmarth Homoeopathic Hospital, Kekri, Dist.Ajmer, Rajasthan (1996), from whom I learned valuable hints in the profession. It was Dr. Mathur who presented me as a famous homoeopath of Delhi in one of his homoepathic camps organized on 18.1.1996 and 19.1.1996 at Kekri. This camp was given a vast publicity through posters and newspapers of Ajmer and Jaipur.

* My thanks to Dr. Satish Sharma, the then Medical officer, (1996) Rajasthan government homoeopathic dispensary, Kekri, Ajmer, from whom I learned a typical method of prescribing in difficult cases of rural population. Many a times, he gave me chance to attend to those difficult cases in government dispensary thus exposing me to a better understanding of homoeopathy. I consider him my worthy guide.

* My hundreds of homoeopathic articles (Hindi and English) published since last ten years in various magazines, newspapers and journals like Vital Informer, Homoeopathic Heritage, Homoeopathy for All, Homoeopathic Sandesh, Vivek Jyoti, Rajasthan Patrika and Dainik Bhaskar are the source of tremendous inspiration for me. The credit for this type of engrossed repertory goes to the editors of magazines, journals and newspapers. I express my sincere thanks to following distinguished and honourable personalities and editors.

* The Editor, Rajasthan Patrika, Jaipur, Rajasthan.

- The Editor, Denik Bhasker, Jaipur, Rajasthan.

- The Editor, Vivek Jyoti, Bhadra, Hanumangarh, Rajasthan.

- Prof. (Dr.) V.K.Gupta, Hony. Editor, HFA, Noida, Former Principal, NHMC, New Delhi and Hony. Advisor to the President of India.

- Dr. Nidhi Luthra, Editor, Homoeopathy for All, Noida.

- Dr. Farokh J. Master, Editor-in-chief, Homoeopathic Heritage, New Delhi.

- Dr. Rohit Jain, Editor, The Homoeopathic Heritage, New Delhi.

- Dr. Manish Bhartiya, Editor, Vital Informer, New Delhi.

- Dr. Sushil Vats, Editor, Vital Informer, New Delhi

- Dr. Hira Singh Namdhari, Ex-editor, Hahnemann Homoeo Sandesh, Vice President, D.H.M.A, New Delhi.

- Dr. V.P.Gupta, Founder, President and managing Editor, Chronicle, S.D.H.A., New Delhi.

Dr. Shiv Dua

Preface . . .

IN THIS era of increased life expectancy of human beings and increasing health disorders inducted by disillusion of modern system of medicine (allopathy), people always look for a safer and effective alternative. Homoeopathy is one of the best safe therapies, which has definite potential. Homoeopathic doctors are mostly practicing in cities and towns. They are not seen in villages except in some regions of West Bengal, Bihar, Rajasthan and Assam. This book is meant for inhabitants of villages and small towns where homoeopaths are not available but some people take interest in homoeopathy and use homoeopathic medicines at their homes. A layman can benefit by self- prescribing with the help of this book irrespective of living in urban and rural background.

The **first part of the book** deals with introduction to homoeopathy in the simplest manner with health attitudes and list of common medicines to be stored at home.

The real utility of this book rests with the **second part**, which has been designed to make a disease-wise diagnosis. There are three basic medicines given here which is to be inducted one after the other in the order of given preference. Keynote has been suggested to refer to first, second and third remedies. When the first fails, the second remedy is to be taken and when the second fails, the third remedy is to be taken. No symptom of the remedy has been given. Only name of disease like cold, fever, cough etc. makes it easy to opt for the remedies in the order given and this will not confuse a layman. If all the three remedies are not found useful, it is better to consult a homoeopath, although its possibility is rare.

BHMS students and the persons, who have knowledge about homoeopathy and understand names of diseases and the symptoms, can switch over to **third part of the book** for single remedy prescription.

In the beginning of disease, there is introduction to the

disease under the column **'Know about ....?'** If it is fever, you will find 'know about fever'. What are fevers, their causes, and their management; how it is to be dealt with? is described here. Then there is a second heading, **'First step treatment'** under which precautions and step wise treatment is suggested.

Every person possesses some skill. All are gifted with some in- built quality, which needs exposure. Those who do not know how to implement skills into practice can benefit from this book. Becoming doctor, engineer or CA are some of desires of children today and their parents show them these dreams. A child does not know much about other professions but his/her visits to doctors fascinate some children. Doctor is the one of the inspirations for the child. Toy- kits containing thermometer, stethoscope, injection and a box of medicines are fancy items for children to enact as a doctor. Some children cultivate a hidden urge to learn medicines but destiny make them company executives, engineers, scientists, chartered accountants, lawyers, chemists, teachers, actors, writers, shop keepers, company secretaries and government servants. Such people can learn homoeopathy through this book for self treatment and treatment of their family. **This book will fulfill their heart-felt desire to cure their friends, relatives and the poor.**

The urge of learning is not limited to non-medical persons. It is a process hidden in every interested person, can be a qualified doctor of allopathic system of medicine. Here is an example as to how learning attains near perfection. I was posted for some days in Lakhasar village of district Bikaner, Rajasthan in connection with Potash investigations in 1976. I stayed with my colleague, Mr. R.M.Singh, Drilling Engineer who was incharge of operation. He had a fast friend, Dr. Sharma who was Medical Officer in government dispensary, Lakhasar. He had completed his MBBS and MS and his posting was in this rural area. Dr. Sharma was at a loss to understand how a homoeopathic medicine without actual medicinal substance could heal? We discussed about it for hours everyday. To know more about it, I gave Dr. Sharma a book to read. I still remember it was 'Beginners guide to Homoeopathy' by T.S. Iyyer. Dr. Sharma read the book a number of times. He was so much convinced about the principles of homoeopathy that he purchased many other books on homoeopathy for study. He further tested homoeopathic medicines on his patients, especially in surgical cases. Time went by and I got transferred to other states of India from time to time. I returned to Bikaner area after 14 years on a posting near Palana and happened to meet Dr. Sharma. I was surprised to know that Dr. Sharma had gained tremendous popularity as a noble surgeon in Bikaner, not merely because of his allopathic practice but by dint of his applying homoeopathy in difficult surgical cases. His services were even sought by the then Chief Minister of Rajasthan, Honourable Shri Bhairon Singh Shekhawat, now Honourable Vice President of India. Here was a glaring example of excellence of homoeopathy.

Homoeopathic prescribing is not that simple but an attempt has been made in this book to make it look like simple. Single remedy given in this book may become a 'hit' or a 'miss' but I am confident that 'hit' will be more than 'miss'. This book is a catalogue with which day to day ailments can be resolved at home. The medicines mentioned in the book need not require any doctor's advise and cannot harm your health, if taken as per directions given on the first page of the book.

Learning any art and science is not difficult, if one takes interest. When grass can grow from cemented brick wall, why learners cannot achieve success and help themselves. This book will be a boon for them.

Dr. Shiv Dua
Faridabad

Contents

PART–I

An Insight   01
Wiser Attitudes for Everyone   07
About Homoeopathy   15
Guidelines for a good Home Kit   23
Uses of Common Remedies at a Glance   33
Injury and Homoeopathy   35

PART–II

Symptoms with Three main Remedies   41

PART–III

According to Symptoms Single Remedy Prescription   67

A

Acne   68
Abdomen pains   69
Allergic to and food aggravations   71
Appetite, Loss of or anorexia   74
Arthritis, gout, rheumatism, joints pains   76
Aversions   80
Awkward behaviour (Mind)   81

B

Backache   83
Bad offensive breath (Halitosis)   86
Bloating of stomach   88
Burns   89
Boils   91

C

Cervical spondylosis	93
Children disorders	93
Colic of babies	99
Common colds (Coryza)	101
Constipation	104
Cough	105
Cramps in legs	109
Cravings (Desires)	111

D

Dandruff	112
Diarrhoea	114
Directional and diagonal diseases	117
Debility or weakness	118

E

Earache or ear pain	118

F

Fever Simple	120
Flatulence (gas)	123

G

Gums disorders	125
Gallbladder disease	127

H

Headaches	129
Hypertension or high blood pressure	131

I

Itching	133
Indigestion	135

Insect bites 137

L

Leucorrhoea 138

M

Menses problems 140
Menopause problems 146
Migraine 147
Mouth ulcers 149

N

Neck pain, cervical spondylosis 151
Numbness 154
Nails, affections of 155
Nausea (Vomiting) 157
Nose bleeding 159

O

Obesity or overweight 160
Operation after effects 164
Opposite symptoms and remedies 165

P

Piles (Haemorrhoids) 168
Prostate gland disease 171

S

Sore throat 173
Snoring 175
Styes (Eruption on the margin of eyes) 177

T

Toothache 178

U

Urinary tract infection (U.T.I) 182

V

Voice disorders, hoarseness   183
Varicose veins   185

W

Warts   187

Tips for success   189
Bibliography   195

Part – I

An Insight

CONGRATULATIONS ! You have purchased this book. This means you care about your health and the health of your family, relatives and friends. You might not be a doctor but you wish to have knowledge about medicines, which should heal avert diseases and should be free of reactions. I can assure one thing, that when your prescribed medicines will cure the patient, you will feel a sense of self-esteem, an elevation of spirits, an eternal ethical satisfaction and a feeling that you have helped someone.

Medicines and potency written in this book will have no adverse effect on your health. It will show no side effects, but if you feel that the medicine has reacted, consult a doctor. Feelings are always variable in different persons. For doubts and feelings, there is no cure. In most of the cases, the homoeopathic medicines written in this book would not bring forth any reactions provided the doses and the potency of the medicines are taken according to the rules laid down thereof.

By taking homoeopathic medicines, you will be nearer to natural health. Health is not a distant dream to achieve in Indian style of living provided you are conscious about maintaining it. Health is a wonderful gift of Almighty instilled through heredity.

Your diet, your life-style, your environment and housing are by dint of the region, you live in; the religion, you belong to, are important for accounting health.

India has variable atmospheric, social and geographical difference in each state. People in each state have different social and climatic environment, different styles of living, different tastes, different diets and different clothes to wear and above all, different way of thinking to tackle health problems. All this has bearing with your health. If the traditional diet, traditional type of housing and traditional life style is not discarded in the region and religion you live in, the best of health is yours. Once you depart from the basics of your traditions, you are moving towards disorders. Your body is tuned to your type of atmosphere and life style at your birth-place and deviation from this is like parting away from mother earth and the normal health. An example is given here. A Bengali friend of mine shifted from his village in Bengal to Delhi on a job appointment. Shifting from a pure healthy atmosphere to polluted city made difference in the health of all his family members, but somehow they continued on taking medicines for minor ills off and on for years. One day, we met after a long time and he explained his health—woes especially skin diseases in all the members of his family. On enquiry, I came to know that he had changed his cooking oil from mustard oil to sunflower oil, thinking it good for blood pressure. On my instance, he changed his cooking oil to mustard oil, and all the skin ailments were gone. When some patients have the same type of ailment in one or more members of family, do enquire about the change of cooking oil. **Our ancestors have been using traditional oils like 'Desi Ghee', mustard oil, groundnut oil, til oil, and coconut oil.** These oils make hereditary constitution and change in the oils can bring metabolic disturbances. Think over this aspect of health.

Treating a disorder at home with the help of homoeopathy is not difficult, provided you have passion to learn.

Homoeopathy has been dealt with in this book in a non-medical method so that you are not confused. The aim of the book is not to make you a doctor but a *keen observer of health*. Once you cure the patients, you will gain tremendous confidence in yourself.

It is my belief that even without help from any system of medicines including homoeopathy, disorders like simple fever, constipation, diarrhoea, cold, cough, headache etc. can be treated at home without medicines through change of diet, routines and simple precautions. The only lacuna is that we lack patience to wait. Everyone desires to get well sooner so that office, study or business does not hamper. To get quick recovery, people take allopathic medicines purchased from the chemist without consulting a doctor. This is dangerous practice for health.

Switching over to homoeopathy is a better alternative than experiencing the hazards of self allopathic-medication. Here below is better alternative of allopathic pain killers in homoeopathy. Try these to see the results by yourself.

HOMOEOPATHIC PAIN KILLERS-I

Upon a severe headache or any other pains, people (mostly in rural India) today purchase tablets known as "Hara patta". In urban India, people know many brands of painkillers. Now try this homoeopathic painkiller. Take Belladonna 30, four pills, every 5 minutes, six doses in thirty minutes and see the results. You will have quick relief. If the pain stops after first, second or any consequent dose, stop further taking the medicine.

HOMOEOPATHIC PAIN KILLERS-II

When Belladonna taken as per above procedure fails, take Magnesium Phos. 6x, 4 tablets, every 5 minutes, four doses in twenty minutes with lukewarm water and you will have wonderful curing results, better than aspirin.

THREE BASIC RULES FOR GOOD HEALTH

The modern medical science in western countries has now realized that Indian system of life-style and diet has a vital role in establishing good health. Here are three gems of health:

- A regular and good diet.

- A regular routine of exercise.

- A regular diversion of thoughts to avoid stress.

A diet taken at home is the best, whatever may be the region or state, you are living in. Make it regular so that it is taken in time. Snatch some time out of your routine to do some exercise daily.

Devote some time for prayers to God at home or make a routine to visit a *temple, Gurudwara, Masjid* or *Church* according to your belief to ward off stress. Open up, discuss and reveal your woes to your partner, friend, or relative and feel secured that there is someone who cares for you and hears you patiently.

HEALTHY LIFE : SOME TIPS

Living in a house can make you healthy or sick depending upon the way you live, the way you adopt to clean it and the way you maintain it. Generally people leave this aspect of cleaning etc. to the ladies of the house and they do not bother to help them. Well, that is the life style men have been told to adopt in India but a lot depends upon male members of the family to select a house, which has following occupancy orders:

- The house should be kept clean and everyday some time should be spent for its upkeep.

- The house should have a definite system of ventilation so that air is received and released in plenty, in the house. If persons living in the house get fresh air, they are likely to live long.

- Do not allow smoking in the house even if you have friends or relatives who smoke, request them to spoil their lungs outside the house. If you happen to be a smoker, better go out of house to destroy yourself. Why should your family members suffer from the ills, you want to induct through passive method.

- If you have some space to accommodate some plants and flowers in the premises of your house, think that you are on way to good health. House—plants keep the air fresh and absorb many toxic chemicals in the air.

- Ensure that all your rooms have adequate natural light system. If you do not have entry for sunlight in your room, make artificial light available in the room. Spend most of your time outside the room either in varandah or other room where natural light is available.

- No one in the family should be allowed to play sound-systems at a higher volume except on certain days of celebrations.

- If you have a computer, microwave system or a television at your home, do not allow your children or other members of family to sit near, on the sides or on the back of TV, microwave or computer. Keep a reasonable distance from these gadgets, when they are operated. Try to spend minimum of time for work on computers.

- Perfumes, pesticides, drain cleaners, floor cleaners, DDT powder, sprays to kill mosquitoes and other domestic chemicals should be kept away from the reach of children.

- All electrical connections, boards and plugs etc., should be installed at a reasonable height on the wall so that children cannot reach them easily. Power point holes on the electric boards near the floor level should be either plugged in or plastic tape should be applied on the holes so that children cannot bore them with their little fingers. Keep children away when using electric press, grinder and washing machine.

● Using heaters in the room during winter is risky for health, if it is turned on too high. At moderate speed, it is smoothening.

● Try not to touch electric switches with wet hands, when in bathroom or kitchen. Wear a rubber shoe in kitchen and bathroom and wipe your hands before switching on or off.

● Do not drink alcohol in the presence of children and do not allow your friends or relatives to drink in presence of children.

● Install a medicine box on a wall in your house. Besides first aid medicines (both allopathic and homoeopathic as suggested in this book), this box should have a separate chamber for hot-water bottle or heat-pad, thermometer, sterile cotton, gauze bandages, surgical adhesive tape and bandages, scissors and tweezer to extract splinters, bee-stings or broken glass pieces.

● Your refrigerator should keep limited quantity of vegetables to be used, say for two days. Do not store vegetables and fruits for more than two days. Make it a practice. Store drinking water in the earthen pot than in the bottles kept in the fridge. Even if you want to drink very cold water, you will not be getting it ready to use if you are not storing it in bottles and in the fridge. You will have to take out ice to make it cool.

Wiser Attitudes
for Everyone

'**I AM** Gyan Budhiraja. He is my friend Narain Das Nagpal'
'My name is Jeewan Das Rawal, pleased to meet both of you.'
'I am Prem Rawal."

What do you conclude? They are dual persons introducing each other.

Yes, they are physically dual entities. Now consider the construction of their bodies irrespective of their identification through name. They are one. Entire human world has one type of structure so far as the body is concerned. The body is made of an enormous complicated structures made of flesh, bones and organs. The varied organs of body are grouped together into different systems and they perform specific body functions. They have minute trillions of body cells, which are the basic components of all the organs and tissues. All the body is compressed into one unit and given identification, a name.

If Budhiraja is suffering from acute bouts of dyspepsia, this means that his digestive system is not functioning properly. If Nagpal suffers from cold and cough, this means that his respiratory system is not in order. These are two examples but there are hundreds of other ailments against which different systems of the body show their discomfort. The causation for an unhealthy body differs from person to person and this may be acquired by infections, pollutions, allergies and improper assimilation or even inherited modality. The causation of a sick body is also due to external accidents and traumas. The wonderful aspect of the body is that it has its own capability to cure and restore the health in minor ailments, leave aside the external injuries. This capability of body is called 'Vital force' in homoeopathy. Every one has his quota of vital force in the body and it is upto the individual to maintain and enhance it through only one mean and that is his attitudes towards his diet, life-style and maintenance through exercises. I name these attitudes as *'Wiser Attitudes'*. Once you know and identify these wiser attitudes, you have capacity to fight diseases and prevent diseases.

Absolute health is not existing now-a-days and it is because of polluted environmental influence, unhygienic mode of living, inherited ailments, drug abuses and ignorance of rules of maintaining good health on the part of people. It can be said that seventy to eighty percent dependence should be on the correct mode of life-style, one leads. This will account for normal health if not absolute health. The rest twenty to thirty percent dependence can be made on treatment by medicines. Body is designed to conserve energy or its vital force provided its maintenence is correct. We have a system of security against diseases. Let this system or health-rule be implemented. The health rules are getting up early in the morning, avoid late night sleeping, going for a walk in the morning, conduct some exercises, take balanced and nutritious diet and avoid excesses in every mode, be it food, sleep, sex, worry, tensions and so on. This has not been possible for most of us to adhere to these golden rules. **The word 'very' is troubling us at every step of life. We are 'very' busy, the life is 'very' speedy, the time is 'very' short and we want to get 'very' rich overnight.**

Having no time and very busy, we opt for ready made food called 'fast food', tin-stuff and variety of junkfood, smashing and storming the market. Our attitude towards simple but nutritious food is totally changed. We know we are eating bad stuff and still we cannot avoid it. We know that cold drinks, so called soft drinks are hard for our body system but still we go on consuming it. I can not compel you to leave all this but can surely suggest some of golden rules and attitudes which will keep you fit inspite of being 'very busy'. **You have no time for morning and evening walks or even light exercises.** For you and the persons of your type, here are some useful suggestions:

- Get up from your bed as per your scheduled time. Do not jump out of bed in a hurry. Sit on the bed with your feet touching the floor. Bring your hands before you, see your palms, rub them together for twenty times and then sweep your face with palms upside down. Repeat this act thrice. Now thank God that you had a nice sleep and that you are found living in this world after your death last night. Every morning God blesses you with a new life to start, with a new morning to resume your work. Sleep, you must agree, is like temporary death. So, take maximum benefit of this new day. (Purpose: By rubbing palms and giving time to your body after sleep, actually you have given time to your heart to cope up with circulation activities ahead for heart to exert; As the heart was at rest during sleep.)

- Drink at least two glasses of water without rinsing your mouth. It is better if the water kept for drinking in the morning is stored in a copper vessel, the previous night. Switch on radio or tape-recorder to listen to devotional songs in praise of God. Walk around the room for a few minutes and go to toilet. (Purpose: Preventing constipation, building self-confidence and enhancing mental power).

- Prefer Indian style seat for evacuation. Defecate with ease without straining. During the act of evacuation, clutch your upper and lower teeth together keeping the mouth closed. This will strengthen the roots of your teeth. If you have a feeling that your bowel is not getting cleared, there are two methods, which you can try. Press thumbs of your both hands against the skin below corners of lower lip. Continue pressure till you count twenty. Release the pressure and count ten. Repeat this act of pressing and releasing thrice. If this method does not work, try another. Put your both hands on your feet so that the palms are pressing them. In this position, raise your buttocks upwards slowly to an extent that your calves and thighs make an angle of ninety or more. While raising the buttocks, take a deep breathing inside. Hold the breath for a while when your buttocks are in raised position and then release the breath out slowly as you lower down your hips. Repeat this act twice or thrice and you will have an easy evacuation.

- Brush your teeth for which keep two brands of toothpastes, one of which should have herbal contents. Use one paste daily for three days and then change to next paste for next three days. Use them one by one and on the seventh day, clean your teeth with 'Datun', if available. If it is not available, use a powder 'Dant-manjan' or salt with mustard oil. Always replace the toothbrush as and when it gets worn out. Sweep your tongue with a tongue-cleaner after brushing.

- Go for a bath. Warm water may be used in winter but immediately after the bath, avoid exposure to cold winds. In summer, try to take a bath in the open instead of a closed bathroom, if you are a male. Taking bath in the open has a freshness that cannot be obtained in closed bathroom.

- Before bath, conduct following activities:

  Go for urination to empty your bladder.

  Smear your right hand index finger with mustard oil and insert it in your umbilical opening ('Nabhi' in Hindi) two to three times so that 'Nabhi' is oiled.

  Now smear your little fingers of both hands with oil and insert them in your ears so that the oil is applied on its inner walls. Do not pour oil in your ears.

Similarly, with the help of right index finger, smear oil in both nostrils of nose.

With the help of left hand index finger, oil your anus, inside of it and the orifice. Wash your hands and now apply some oil on both of the great toes.

(Purpose: Strenghening the intestines, preventing ears and nose from pollution-diseases, precaution against piles and other rectum diseases and taking care of eye-sight by lubricating your great toes).

- During bathing fill your mouth with water so that your cheeks appear swollen with water inside. Hold this water in the mouth till you finish the bath. Apply soap only twice a week. Instead rub your body with your hands and go on pouring water. After the bath, with the help of a mug full of water, splash the water on your closed eyes for at least ten times. Open the eyes and splash water on your opened eyes only once. During this splashing, your mouth is full of water, which you had put before starting the bath. After splashing of water, release the water from your mouth now. Wipe your body with a soft towel vigoursly after the bath. (Purpose: Care of eyes, face and skin).

- If you have a prayer-place at home, devote two to five minutes in prayers and light 'dhoop' or 'agarbatti'. Your food and dress is the next thing. After breakfast, rinse your mouth with water for five times so that all food particles are removed. This should be done after lunch and dinner also. The best way is to keep the water in mouth and rub the teeth/gums with the help of your index finger. Use of toothpick after a meal is a healthy habit.

- Come out of your home, take deep breathing three times inhaling and exhaling to get fresh air, look back at your sweet home and bid goodbye to your family. You are now entering a world of pollutions.

- If your work involves lot of sitting on the chair, try to change your sitting postures every half an hour of continuous work or leaning on the table. Slip to left, to right, forward and backward on the chair. Tilt and stretch your back and neck from time to time. Stretch your legs straight, move your neck sidewise and forward and backward and cover your eyes with your cupped palms for a while.

- Returning home at the dinner table, chew your food in such a way that it becomes a paste in your mouth and your intestines have an easy job to digest it. Do not watch TV and prefer not to talk much during the dinner-time. After dinner, go to toilet to empty your bladder (urination). Return and sit erect on your calves, folding your legs beneath the hips and placing your palms on the thighs. Sit in this posture for fifteen minutes.

- Before going to bed, wash your face, hands and feet. Thank God that you had a good day. (Be it otherwise, always think positive). Do not cover your face with blanket or quilt in winter. Instead of this you can wear a cap, if required.

- Eat whatever is your routine but make sure that you eat one 'Roti' or a little rice less than you desire to eat.

- Drink water half an hour before or after taking meals. If you cannot resist taking water during meals, you can have half a glass of water in mid of meals.

- Try to make a habit of clamping your upper and lower teeth together during the act of urination.

- Do not insert sticks in your ears to clear wax. Do not insert fingers in your nostrils frequently. Instead of this, you can clean your nose by using handkerchief.

- If you have one time stool habit in the morning, try to attempt defecation in the evening also. Wash the anus with your left hand thoroughly with plenty of water and never use warm or hot water for this purpose in winter.

Include the above attitudes in your life routine. This will not take much of time, of which you are so short of, being a busy man or woman. This type of routine will not have extra burden on your living style but this will help you fight invasions of disorders or diseases in your body. You have no time for exercise, no time to get up early in the morning or go to bed early. You return from office or business meeting late at night and cannot have walks after dinner. If you adopt above rituals, you will feel secured against disorders of your vital organs. I do not feel that I should strongly profess about it. A trial by you for a few days will show results. No one is free from external infections and polluted atmosphere and if these envelope you, better to consult a doctor immediately.

About Homoeopathy

THIS BOOK is related to homoeopathy and hence it is not out of way to state something about its fundamentals and uses so that it proves beneficial for the readers. Homoeopathy is a system of medicine or a therapy meant to maintain or restore normal health through specific therapeutic agents made according to certain scientific principles.

The word 'Homoeopathy' is taken from the Greek and the meaning is 'similar suffering'. The principle that works in homoeopathy is *'like cures like'*. This can be illustrated in a simple way. If a medicinal substance can produce the symptoms of sickness when it is taken in large quantity, it has also the power to heal the same symptoms when taken in infinitesimally small quantity. Homoeopathy has proved to do so without any harm to the body or without any side effects.

It was Hippocrates, the father of medicine (470-400 BC) who developed a concept that there are only two methods of healing, 'The contraries' and 'The similars'. The contrary is when a poison is nullified by an agent opposing poison whereas the similar is when a case of poison is healed by the use of same poison as healing agent. Hippocrates also wrote that every disease has its own nature and arises from external causes, from the cold, from the sun, from the changing winds or seasons and that our *nature is the physician of all diseases*. After

Hippocrates came Paracelsus (1493-1541) who believed in the harmony of the whole universe and advocated that poison that causes a disease should also act as medicine to cure. He supported the theory of 'similars' of Hippocrates. This was another way of expression of the theory, 'like cures like'.

In time to come, there was Dr. Samuel Hahnemann (1755-1843) who founded the principle of homoeopathy based upon the theory of similars. He was not only a doctor but a chemist and a linguist too. He termed this phenomenon of like cures like as 'similia similibus curentur'. By this term he meant that in order to cure disease, we must seek medicines that can excite similar symptoms in the healthy body. He wrote this finding in a book called 'The Organon of Rational Art of Healing' or 'the Organon of healing art', which ran into six editions, each one modified and expanded. One can judge the popularity of homoeopathic system of medicine by number of editions of the book, in the era when controversies and opposing forces due to trade jealousy were in great strength. A discovery is not easy to be gained on grounds.

Hahnemann believed that there is a balancing mechanism in our body that keeps us healthy. This balancing mechanism is called 'vital force', an energetic substance, which has no physical or chemical identity in the body and still it works in our body and literally gives life to us. Vital force or the balancing mechanism can also be termed as 'defence mechanism' of body. This is another method of referring to vital force, which the modern doctors call immune system. Hahnemann believed that diseases attack only when vital force is weak. Homoeopathic medicines act as catalyst to re-energise the body through its gentle stimulation. It is unlike suppressing the disease by medicines of the orthodox system.

Homoeopathy believes that body heals by itself provided it is cared for and properly fed. The homoeopathic medicines stimulate the power of self-healing and a body is taken as a whole without bothering for the name of disease. For every person there is different medicine although he may be suffering from simple fever. It is the symptoms that are taken and then a medicine is selected that should have capability of producing same symptoms. Normally one medicine is selected and a minimum dose is given. It is not only the symptoms of the disease that help a homoeopath for selection of a remedy but a history of patient is also taken. Patient's diseases in the past, history of diseases of his or her parents, his personality, behaviour, temperament, liking, disliking and his constitution etc. are also taken into account before arriving at a remedy. So, taking up a case in homoeopathy is a serious affair and once it is undertaken as per the exact laid down norms, the results are always positive. The remedy selected as per the totality of symptoms is bound to reflect cure, smoothly and sooner. This book does not deal with long process of case taking. You are not a doctor and hence your dealing with the medicines is different and exactly according to the name of disease. For example if you suffer from headache, you have to see the title headache, check the symptoms given against each medicine and take the medicine.

A FEW FUNDAMENTALS CONCEIVED BY THE FOUNDER OF HOMOEOPATHY (FROM HIS BOOK 'THE ORGANON OF MEDICINE')

- The first and sole duty of the physician is to restore health.

- The ideal cure consists in restoring health in a prompt, mild and permanent manner, by removing and annihilating disease by the shortest, safest and most certain means based upon principles that are simple and intelligent.

- The physician must be able to recognize the body in normal health and in disease.

- The physician should be able to judge the curative indication in each disease.

- The physician should be well acquainted with the healing (therapeutic) effect of medicines.

- The disease is to be assessed by symptoms. A symptom is expression of change or disturbance in a healthy body produced by some morbid agent.

- The knowledge of a medicine's action should be obtained by experimentation on the healthy human body.

- The relation between the above two points (knowledge of medicines and symptoms) is by the principle, 'Like cures like".

- The remedy selected should be given singly, not combined with any other medicine.

- The dose of the selected remedy should be the smallest dose that will cure, hence the minimum dose.

- The method of selection of remedy is on totality of symptoms.

- The totality of symptom is symptoms observed in a patient (both subjective and objective) and the symptoms should bear the closest similitude to the symptoms of the medicine.

The Physician must know:

- What is curable in a disease?

- What modality may best cure or alleviate a particular disease?

- The precise indications for the remedy.

- The effective duration of its effects.

- When to repeat the remedy, when to stop it, and when to change the remedy?

PHARMACY IN HOMOEOPATHY

Homoeopathic medicines are prepared from a variety of sources, the vegetation, the animals, the minerals and even venoms. The medicines from these sources are made according to the specifications of the homoeopathic pharmacopoeia. Although given in small doses, they are effective, gentle and safe.

Medicines are prepared in a code depicting their strength, which is called *potentisation*. Diluting and shaking the medicinal substance by turn until molecules of the original substance are no more left in the liquid, achieve potentisation. The potentised liquid is given a number, 'C' or 'X' according to method of dilution. If the medicine that you are taking has a code of 30 C, this means that the process of diluting and shaking has taken place for thirty times, starting with one part of crude drug diluted with ninety nine parts of alcohol each time. The first such dilution is 1 C. From 1 C dilution one drop is taken and diluted with ninety nine drops of alcohol. The outcome is 2 C. The procedure goes on. *More dilute is the substance; stronger is its effect.* If the medicine that you are taking has a code of 6 X, the dilutions are made starting with one drop of drug with nine drops of alcohol each time. A suffix of 30 C or 30 with the name of medicine is one and the same thing.

The medicines are available in the market in pills, powder and liquid. It is better for the readers of this book and learners to purchase medicine in pills of size 30. Homoeopathic pills are sweet because they contain milk sugar (lactose). These pills are converted into medicines by mixing some drops of liquid-potentised medicine.

The purpose of this book is not to go deep into the subject and also avoid all technical or complicated medicinal words. If you are interested in deep and systematic study of homoeopathy, many books are available with the publishers of this book.

DO'S AND DONT'S FOR TAKING MEDICINES

- In order not to confuse the reader, who is supposed to take the medicine without consulting the doctor, it is suggested that the medicine prescribed against each disease be taken four times a day with minimum interval of three hours.

- The medicine should be taken in the dose of 4 pills at a time. The pills size to be obtained from the chemist is 30. Please see the method of preparing medicines on page 25 of this book.

- To get better results, it is advised that nothing should be taken 15 minutes before taking the medicine and 15 minutes after taking the medicine.

- Take the medicine on tongue and suck it. It will dissolve itself. Do not chew it. No preventions like taking garlic, onions, coffee etc. are required as was the regime or rule with homoeopathy in the past. Some homoeopaths' prefer that the medicines should be placed under the tongue and not on the tongue. It is one and the same.

- However, precautions like taking light diet in indigestion, fever, diarrhoea or constipation and avoiding curds in coughs etc. have to be taken.

- When the complaints for which you have taken medicine subside, you can stop taking medicine. If the symptoms return, start taking the medicine again. If there is no improvement in your acute illness after 24 hours, choose another medicine according to changed symptoms, if any, or consult a doctor.

- If there is no significant change in the health condition after taking eight doses of medicine, consider that the remedy, you have selected is wrong. Select the next one. If this also does not work, consult a doctor. Tell the doctor about the medicines you had been taking for the symptoms.

- Medicines should be purchased from reliable firms and should be stored in places free from dust, smoke, sun ray's, strong smells and away from allopathic drugs, tinctures, iodex, camphor, essences and perfumes. Try not to burn incense in the room where you store medicines. Keep the medicines in a wooden/ steel box or cupboard.

- The best time for use of medicines is early in the morning on empty stomach, if not otherwise mentioned with the medicine.

- In the case of fevers, medicines should be taken when the temperature is coming down.

- In case of diarrhoea or vomiting, the medicine should be taken after evacuation or vomiting.

- Chewing of tobacco, smoking or taking 'Paan' is forbidden one hour before and one hour after the time when medicine is taken.

DIFFERENCE BETWEEN ACUTE AND CHRONIC DISEASE

One must realize the difference between acute and chronic disease before taking homoeopathic medicines. This book is dealing with day-to-day acute diseases or disorders and not with chronic diseases like diabetes, asthma, tuberculosis etc. It should be made a rule not to treat a patient whose disease is not understood and is of long standing. For such patients, doctor's consultation is necessary. Cold, coryza, cough, flu, diarrhoea, simple constipation, food poisoning, chicken pox and simple fever etc. are acute diseases. The remedies selected from this book will soon cure the cases. Acute disease is having a limited course and it is not deep seated. In most of the cases, acute disease will clear itself. Acute disease has three stages:

I.   **The period of onset or incubation period.** There are not much of symptoms of disease in this period.

II. The second period is when symptoms of disease appear. This stage is called **acute phase.**

III. When the patient gets cured and feels improved, this stage is called **convalescent phase.**

Acute disease is one in which some virus or disease germs enter the body and having passed through the prodrome (fore runner), progressive and decline phases, are extruded out of the body as we see in measles.

Chronic disease shows the permanent entry of one of the three fundamental miasms, Psora, Syphilis or Sycosis. It has a continuous progressive tendency with no inclination to recovery soon. Let us not worry about the term miasms* [Miasms are the names given to a group of diseases. When Hahnemann was investigating the truth about homoeopathy, he was surprised to find that some of his patients did not respond to the well-selected constitutional remedies and some patients did give response but their improvement was short lived. The disease relapsed after a short time. He took pains to collect data of all those patients along with their family history of diseases. He concluded after a long experimentation that 'those diseases' constitute some 'blocks' that stopped the constitutional remedies to make improvement in health. Hahnemann called these 'blocks' as 'miasms' and developed a comprehensive but complex theory on miasms. In order to make evaluation of these miasms, homoeopaths assess them through history of patient, both inherited and acquired, their constitutional strength and personal family background.] here in this book, which is meant for beginners.

Chronic diseases are deep-seated. They develop slowly and continue for a longer period and make the condition of patient deteriorated in general health. There is no prediction as to how long it will take to cure and how much time will it last.

––––––––––––––––––

Guidelines for a Good Home Kit

METHOD OF PREPARING MEDICINE

- Acquire following medicines from a good and reliable medical store.

- All medicines should be in dilution and in 30th potency, packed in 1 drahm bottle with a dropper on it.

- Purchase one packet of globules no. 30, say 200 gms and also about 50 empty 1 drahm bottles.

- To prepare medicine for use, fill the bottle with globules and pour 7 to 8 drops of dilution of required medicine in it. Close the cork or lid and shake it well so that the medicine wets all the globles in the bottle. To avoid confusion about shaking the bottle, you can enquire from the chemist when purchasing medicines. He will guide you about how to prepare medicine.

- 200 potency medicines can be purchased from the market when you learn the use of single medicine and when you have read the third part of the book.

SOME COMMONLY USED REMEDIES
AND THEIR GENERAL USE

1. **Aconitum napellus:** Effects of fear, exposure to cold air, sore throat, sudden high fever, dry cough in children, restlessness.

2. **Antimonium crudum:** Complaints from over-eating, cracks on corners of mouth and nostril, lips dry, corns on soles, diarrhoea alternates with constipation, tongue white coated, vomiting of bile, curdled milk, indigestion, empty bleching, tasting of food just taken, for people who are gluttons who eat more than they need.

3. **Allium cepa:** Common colds, sneezing and eyes watering. Nasal discharge irritates but watering from eyes do not cause irritation. Sore throat with burning.

4. **Apis mellifica:** Insect bites, burning pains and swollen ankles, symptoms relieved by cold compresses or cool air, urticaria.

5. **Argentum nitricum:** Acidity, dyspepsia, mental strain, laryngitis, headache.

6. **Arnica montana:** Injuries without bleeding, bruises, shocks from injury, before dental treatment or surgery, exhaustion.

7. **Arsenicum album:** Diarrhoea, vomiting, food poisoning, hay fever (colds), abdomen and stomach cramps, symptoms relieved by warmth and sips of cold water, restlessness and weakness.

8. **Belladonna:** Throbbing pains, high fever that comes on suddenly, dry skin burning, throbbing pains in the head, oversensitive to light, facial neuralgia, mumps, sore throat, measles.

9. **Bryonia alba:** Muscular pains, chest pains due to colds, dry painful coughs relieved by holding chest, fever develops slowly, extreme thirst for large

quantities of water, symptoms worse by slight motion, desire to be left alone.

10. **Calcarea carbonica:** Anaemia, complaints from getting wet, catches cold easily, profuse menses, acne, cramps, appetite excessive, acidity, constipation.

11. **Calcarea phosphorica:** Severe stomach pains after eating, catches cold easily, complaints from loss of body fluids, dentition, anaemia, brain fag, fractures slow in healing.

12. **Calcarea fluorica:** Cracked joints, thick nasal catarrh, sneezing with difficulty, better for sneezing, pain in lower back, bleeding piles, tooth decay, bones enlargement.

13. **Cantharis vesicatoria:** Burning during urination, burns and scalds before blister formation, pains burning, sunburns, cystitis (desire to urinate, constant, frequent, ineffectual urge, pains before, during and after urination; urine red, hot and scanty).

14. **Carbo vegetabilis:** Indigestion with flatulence, better by passing wind, hair loss, headache, nose bleed, cold sweat, breath smells, loss of body fluids, hoarseness, acne and general debility.

15. **Chamomilla:** Teething infants, nausea, migraine, diarrhoea in children, any sickness relating to children who are having bad temper and irritability.

16. **China officinalis:** Anaemia, appetite lost, complaints from loss of body fluids, painless diarrhoea, exhaustion, flatulence obstructed, stomach bloated, nervous headache.

17. **Cocculus indicus:** Travelling sickness, nausea, mental and physical strain due to loss of sleep, exhaustion, complaints from anger, grief.

18. **Colocynthis:** Main colic remedy, belly bloated and painful, violent gripping pain with diarrhoea, nausea or vomiting, pains better by bending double and passing stool, worse after drinking, cold drinks, before stool and after eating fruits.

19. **Euphrasia officinalis:** Eyes inflammed, watering

eyes with burning, conjunctivitis, measles, nasal cararrh bland watery.

20. **Ferrum phosphoricum:** Nose bleed, hot flushes, varying appetite, fear, debility, first stage of fever, vomiting of undigested food, sour eructations.

21. **Gelsemium sempervirens:** Influenza with weak aching muscles, shivering fever, little thirst, sluggish, onset of complaints slow, anxiety including trembling, measles, examination or interview nervousness, sore throat, runny nose, headache.

22. **Hamamelis virginiana:** Nosebleed aggravation morning time, varicose veins, legs and thighs; heavy periods, bleeding piles (large and sore, especially after child birth or pregnancy).

23. **Hepar sulphuris calcareum:** Catches cold easily, wheezing in chest, sore throat as if something is stuck in throat, harsh dry cough with yellow mucus, and abscesses and boils that would not heal, skin sensitive to touch, sour smelling sweat and coldness.

24. **Hypericum perforatum:** Injuries to nerves, bruising of sensitive areas such as fingers, toes, lips, eyes, ears and coccyx, shooting pain along the nerves.

25. **Ignatia amara:** Shock, bereavement, weeping, hysteria, piercing headaches (especially forehead), grief and sadness following emotional loss, swinging mood, sore throat better swallowing, liquids more difficult to swallow than solids.

26. **Ipecacuanha:** Nausea and vomiting (bile, food, green), whether or not accompanied by other symptoms, constant, morning sickness, nose bleeding, spasmodic wheezing cough with nausea, retching or blue face.

27. **Kalium bichromicum:** Stringy yellow sputum, dry cough, sore throat, nasal catarrh, sticky crusts in nostrils, dry hard to pick out, earache with discharges thick, yellow, smelly, empty sour belching after eating.

28. **Kalium phosphoricum:** Tiredness, exhaustion, indigestion, anaemia, weakness during convalescence and after influenza, mental strains, overwork, depressed.

29. **Ledum palustre:** Rheumatic complaints of joints, skin punctured, cuts and wounds, pains wandering, better cold bathing, bites, stings of insects, black eye due to injury.

30. **Lycopodium clavatum:** Chronic dyspepsia, right sided symptoms worse between 4 PM and 8 PM, pain in lower back, nasal catarrh yellow, nose blocked dry, constipation, desire to pass stool ineffectual, knotty hard stools, cystitis (see its meaning in Cantharis vesicatoria above), hair loss, indigestion (belching; acrid, empty), pre-examination nervousness and stage fright.

31. **Mercurius solubilis:** Complaints from getting chilled, fowl breath, body- odour, diarrhoea, mumps, abscesses of glands and roots of teeth decayed nasal catarrh (bloody, burning, green-yellow), cystitis, earache (discharges blood streaked, smelly), eye inflammation, mouth ulcers, sore throat.

32. **Natrium muriaticum:** Tiredness, exhaustion, confused, depressed, sinus troubles, sneezy colds, running nose, discharge from eyes watery, constipation, stools crumbling like small balls, takes more of common salt, cracks on lips and around mouth.

33. **Nux vomica:** Useful for workaholics who stay out too late, do no exercise, eat rich food, drink alcohol. All sort of disturbances that follow over-indulgence in food, alcohol, coffee or tobacco, all complaints worse in morning, constipation with unfinished feeling, itching piles (due to pregnancy), hangovers, cramping pains in stomach, cystitis, flatulence, bloated abdomen, indigestion .

34. **Phytolacca decandra:** Sore throat, throat dark red,

tonsils swollen-better cold drink, swallowing difficult and causes the pains to shoot through both ears, mouth ulcers, pains appear and disappear suddenly and shoot upwards, breath smells, loss of voice.

35. **Pulsatilla nigricans:** Useful for women as Nux vomica is useful for men. Change of life, gentle, yielding, easily moved to tears or laughter, depressed before menses, irregular menses, indigestion, hay fever, headaches, styes (worse upper lids), thirstless, changeable complaints, earache with thick yellow or green discharge, indigestion (belching tasting of food just eaten, with heartburn), joints pain wandering.

36. **Rhus toxicodendron:** Complaints from getting wet and change of weather, rheumatism, lumbago, sciatica, strains of joints and tendons, herpes of lips, backache with stiffness, aggravation rest and on beginning to move, sore throat, throat tickling and dry, stiff neck due to draughts, getting chilled and over lifting, nervous exhaustion with heaviness and restlessness, urticaria.

37. **Ruta graveolens:** Eye-strain, weak dim eyesight due to too much close work and overstraining eyes, aching and lightness in chest, dislocation and pain in bones, in parts lain on, sore bruised, sprains in hands, ankles, in wrist, tennis elbow.

38. **Sepia officinalis:** Change of life, morning sickness, suppressed or delayed menses, painful periods, backache, cystitis, weakness, hair loss, hot flushes.

39. **Symphytum officinale:** Bone fractures; rheumatic and arthritic conditions leading to bone injuries or fractures.

40. **Silicea terra:** Boils, abscesses of glands, decayed roots of teeth, constipation with ineffectual straining, flatulence with smelly wind, gum boils, headaches

with pain in back of head, chronic headache, sinus problems, sore throat, stitching pains in throat, helps to push out foreign bodies from the skin, toothache with swelling of face and glands.

THERMAL BEHAVIOUR OF REMEDIES

In our country, we are guided by the nature of the eatables. The eatables are either cold or hot in nature. For example, Potatoes are dry and hot in nature, lagenaria siceraria ('Lauki' or 'Kaddu' in Hindi) is moist and cold in nature and radish ('Muli') is both hot and cold in nature. In nature means, when these items are consumed, they will produce their hot or cold (or both) effect on the body. In the same manner, the medicines made out of herbs, vegetables, plants, minerals and animals also carry hot and cold nature.

Human body is not of same nature. It has to be either cold or hot in its capacity of absorption. Some people are very chilly and some do not require much of clothing in winter. Similarly some people need heavy cooling effect and cool air. They perspire heavily during summer but some of us do not perspire much and do not feel that hot. If the medicines are given according to the nature of individuals, they are supposed to act better. Medicines are, therefore, divided into three groups.

- Cold medicines

- Hot medicines

- Both hot and cold medicines

In my practice, I have not been bothering about hot and cold remedies except dealing with chronic cases. **You need not bother about hot and cold remedies at your level of learning and especially when the diseases are of acute nature.** 15 out of 40 medicines given in the above list are both hot and cold in nature (Serial no 1, 2, 5, 6, 8, 9, 14, 15, 25, 26, 29, 30, 31, 32 and 35).

SOME USEFUL OINTMENTS AT HOME
FOR LOCAL APPLICATION

Use of external remedies in homoeopathy is not well proved and not considered truely homoeopathic. The remedies given hereunder are those, which are useful externally in emergency. The external remedies are not potentised and are actually abstracts of herbs/plants. In the market, external remedies of homoeopathy are available in the form of lotions, ointments, tinctures, creams and oils. Following ointments/ mother tinctures are recommended for keeping at home for general use:

1. **Arnica ointment:** Used externally for bruises, sore muscles, sprains, bed sores and corns. Do not use it for open wounds and cuts.

2. **Calendula ointment:** Minor cuts and wounds, rashes, eczema, cracked skin, nappy rash and sun burns. First clean the surface of skin to be sure that no dirt exists and then apply it gently.

3. **Hamamelis ointment:** Piles, varicose veins.

4. **Aesculus ointment:** Piles, varicose veins. If you are taking Hamamelis or Aesculus internally also, prefer to use locally the same. Better to take professional advise for their use because some ointments have mixture of both and are available in the market with brand names.

5. **Hypericum ointment:** Cuts, wounds, cold sores, boils, insect bites, sun burns.

6. **Euphrasia eye drops:** Eyes infection, inflammations, watering of eyes or burning due to dirt.

7. **Ledum ointment:** Insect bites where swelling is prominent, punctured wounds, scratches.

8. **Ruta ointment:** Bruises, sprains, tennis elbow, corns.

9. **Cantharis ointment:** Burns.

10. **Rhus tox ointment:** Joint pains, sprains, and strains.

11. **Urtica ointment:** Intense itching of skin, urticaria, blotches, burns confined to the skin and with no blisters, scalds.

12. **Phytolacca Q:** Use it for sore throat and throat infection. Ten drops of this mother tincture should be put in 100 ml of lukewarm water and then gargled. Purchase 30 ml of this tincture.

Note : Many companies manufacture each of the above ointments or lotions and it has direction for use written over it except Phytolacca.

Uses of Common Remedies at a Glance

DIGESTION PROBLEMS

Nux vomica, Pulsatilla nigricans, Antimonium crudum, Carbo vegitabilis, China officinalis, Lycopodium clavatum, Argentum nitricum, Chamomilla.

BODYACHE

Rhus toxicodendron, Bryonia alba, Kalium Bichromicum, Ruta graveolens, Phytolacca decandra, Calcarea carbonica, Calcarea phosphorica, Colocynthis, Belladonna, Ledum palustre.

COLD, COUGH, CORYZA PROBLEMS

Aconitum napellus, Allium cepa, Gelsemium sempervirens, Arsenicum album.

GENERAL WEAKNESS PROBLEMS

China officinalis, Sepia officinalis, Kalium phosphoricum, Calcarea phosphorica.

INJURY, BONES, WOUNDS PROBLEMS

Arnica montana, Calcarea phosphorica, Calcarea fluorica, Symphytum, Ruta graveolens, Ledum palustre, Hypericum perforatum.

DEPRESSION, GRIEF, WORRY PROBLEMS

Ignatia amara, Natrium muriaticum, Pulsatilla nigricans, Kalium phosphorica, Sepia officinalis.

BOILS, ABSCESSES

Hepar sulphur, Belladonna, Silicea terra, Mercurius solubilis, Arnica montana.

SORE THROAT

Belladonna, Silicea terra, Mercurius solubilis, Phytolacca decandra.

FEVER (SIMPLE)

Aconitum napellus, Belladonna, Ferrum phosphorica, Gelsemium sempervirens, China officinalis.

Note : The above information is for general knowledge and the final selection of medicine should be made from the following chapters, 'disease-wise keynotes', part II and part-III.

Injury and Homoeopathy

IT IS common to see children getting injuries, sportsmen getting sprains and injuries, women getting cuts, burns and injuries in the kitchen work, men getting cuts while shaving. The list of injuries is very long. Everyone gets injured at one time or the other and everyone runs to the doctor for help. If you are a learner and keeping homoeopathic medicines at home, you can act as a doctor and can give first-aid help provided the injury is not of major nature, involving surgery or stitches. Here is a simple ritual you have to follow to get eternal bliss of curing others.

HANDLING MINOR CUTS

Wash the cuts or wound with soap and lukewarm water to clean it and see that there is nothing left inside, especially the dirt, which can penetrate the wound. This dirt debris may cause infection. Now use some antibiotic ointment. This seals the wound with its film and there is no need for bandage. Bandaging of cuts is only needed when the wound is big.

HANDLING BLEEDING AND DEEP CUTS

Control the bleeding first by pressure of your fingers above the wound for some time. It should not be too tight to make the injured person feel discomfort. The decrease in bleeding will indicate the pressure to be applied. Keep the wounded part in an elevated position i.e if the wound is on leg, keep a cushion below leg and remove the pillow from beneath the head so that the legs are elevated above head level. Now place some sterile gauze pads on the wound and keep the pressure over it till blood seeps from it. When the blood stops seeping, tie the bandage over the pad and place some ice on the bandaged dressing. It will constrict the blood vessels further.

If the bleeding does not get controlled in spite of above measure, rush to the doctor. If the child is injured at the torso, cover the wound with sterile dressing, keep a constant pressure over it and carry the child to the doctor.

NON-BLEEDING INJURIES

Arnica montana is the well-known homoeopathic medicine to non-homoeopathic families for its curing qualities in injuries. This medicine has worldwide reputation in the field of homoeopathy like *Calcarea phosphorica* that has earned laurels for dentition problems. Even allopathic doctors prescribe this.

Injuries that are blood-less, in the form of bruises, elevated swelling or where the skin is turned red or blue need four doses of *Arnica montana* 30 in a day. Next day, if the pain and swelling exists, give *Rhus toxicodendron* 30, two doses in a day. Third day, if the pains are gone but weakness exists, a dose of *Calcarea carbonica* 30 will erase all discomforts of injury. If the pain and swelling is less after first day of taking *Arnica montana*, there is no need to take *Rhus toxicodendron* and *Calcarea carbonica*.

BLEEDING INJURIES

For an injury that is bleeding, Ledum palustre 30 is the first medicine to be given in two doses at an interval of 15 minutes. It works like giving anti-tetanus injection. After an hour of this, give Hypericum perforatum 30 in three doses at the interval of two hours each. Needless to say that measures like washing the cuts with fresh water and antiseptic solution and pressing the area of injury to stop bleeding have to be taken. If bleeding is not controlled, consult a doctor. Medicines should be given irrespective of stopping of bleeding or not.

DIFFERENT TYPES OF INJURIES AND DIFFERENT HOMOEOPATHIC MEDICINES

* You are hammering a nail into the wall and by mistake **injured your finger by hammer,** there is no bleeding but severe pang of pain, take *Ledum palustre* 30, three times a day for one day.

* While cutting vegetables with knife, the **finger is cut and there is bleeding,** put your finger under flowing water to stop bleeding and then take *Hypericum perforatum* 30, three times a day for one day.

* When closing the door, **the finger is pressed between the doors;** when rising from the chair, the knee is hurt against table; when moving in the house, the elbow strikes against window or bed; when injury is on the bone and there is no bleeding; under all these conditions, take *Ruta graveolens* 30, three times a day for one day.

* When a **rat has bitten** while sleeping or there is cat or dog bite, take *Ledum palustre* 200 one dose and consult a doctor.

* When the child has **fallen from stairs** and hitted against floor on his back, injuring back and spinal area, give *Hypericum perforatum* 200, one dose irrespective of bleeding or non-bleeding. Then consult a doctor.

* When the **cut on any part of body** is by a machine blade or the injury has not dried after an operation, give *Staphysagria* 200, one dose.

- When children fall during play and get non-bleeding injuries, *Arnica montana* is sufficient. When they fall with hands down on the ground injuring their palms, they get **scratches and slight bleeding.** The medicine for such condition is *Hypericum perforatum* 30, three times a day for one day.

- When injury is due to falling on stones or **by hitting of stones,** the skin is broken. The medicine is *Calendula officinalis* 30, three times a day for one day.

- When a **broken piece of glass** has entered the skin of foot or hand, extract the broken glass from the skin and take *Hypericum perforatum* 30, three times a day for one day. The same is the medicine when there is cut on the face, while shaving.

- When children fight and exchange **slaps and hand-blows hitting** the face of others: when blows leave the skin beneath eyes blue and red; *Arnica montana* 30 is the remedy, three times a day for one day.

- ***Sprain or strain of foot of athletes or children** while playing need Arnica montana 30 for one day, four times a day. Next day, give Bellis perennis 30, three times a day. [Sprain or strain and fracture: Sprain or strain is same while treating. Sprain is tear of ligament (Band of tissues joining bones) and strain is tear of muscles. Fracture is tear of bones. Complete rest and compression are needed in all the cases. The doctor has to be consulted in case of fracture.]

- The first medicine after a major accident like **breaking of bones** is one dose of Arnica montana, 1M. Repeat one more dose after four hours. Later, let orthopaedician do the repairing job now. When plastering has been done and bone binding is needed, give *Symphytum officinale* 200, two doses a day for three days. From fourth day, start *Calcarea phosorica* 6x, four times a day for 10 days. There will be easy and early binding of bones.

- For the **head injuries** of children, Arnica montana 30 is the first remedy when there is bruising and shock. Give it four times a day for two days. When there is weakness and exhaustion after head injury, give *Kalium phosphoricum* 6X three times a day for seven days along with *Arnica montana* 30. When the head has crashed and there is headache and pain in the occiput after a few days of injury, give *Natrium sulphuricum* 30, three times a day for seven days.

- When there are eye traumas, there are bruises or scratches around eyes, give *Arnica montana* 30, two times a day alongwith *Euphrasia officinalis* 30, two times a day for three days. If the eyes get hot, burning and watering, only *Euphrasia officinalis* 30, three times a day for three days. Locally, *Euphrasia eye drops* can be used for better results. If there is blunt injury by hitting of ball, give *Symphytum officinale* 200, two doses at the interval of one hour and if not improved, consult the doctor.

There are wonderful medicines in homoeopathy, which when given before and after a surgical operation, give miraculous results. The patients do not get nervous; feel less of pains and less of after- effects of injections (swelling and tumor at the place of vaccination, vaccinosis). *Bellis perennis, Rhus toxicodendron, Staphysagria* and *Thuja occidentalis* are the medicines, which should be given in consultation with the homoeopath.

How to Identify Fracture?

How to identify whether it is a fracture or not? Generally fractures do not show swelling whereas sprains or strains can be swollen. To see whether a foot ankle has been sprained or fractured, one has to hold the calf at its wider region with both hands and squeeze hard. If pain is felt at the ankle, it may be broken. Of course, X-ray is the best mode of diagnosis.

STORE FOUR MEDICINES AT HOME
FOR COMMON INJURIES

You need not spend more, store only four medicines at home for injuries; Arnica montana 30, Ledum palustre 30, Hypericum perforatum 30 and Ruta graveolens 30, 1 dm each in pills no 30. In case of relief of pains and condition, do not repeat the medicine on the second day. In case of no relief after a day of their uses, consult a homoeopath.

This article is meant for those who have adopted homoeopathy as a hobby, as a favourite pastime and want to learn it as armour of first aid. Tear this page and keep it as a record. In the course of its frequent reading and use of medicines, you will remember the uses of these medicines.

Part – II

Symptoms with Three Main Remedies

GENERAL RULES OF TAKING REMEDIES

- Remedies given against each disease or disorder are in the order of preference. First remedy to be given in the first instance failing which the second and then the third one if the second fails.

- All medicines are to be taken in 30th potency.

- 4 pills make a dose.

- The size of pills considered here is 30.

- Four doses are to be taken in a day at an interval of 3 hours (12 hours).

- In severe pains, the remedy can be repeated every ten minutes with limitation of 3 doses.

- When there is no relief after taking the first medicine for 24 hours (eight doses), change to the second remedy and consequently to third remedy finding no relief by again eight doses.

- When there is no relief even after taking all the three medicines turn by turn, consult a homoeopath.

- When there is partial relief in symptoms, continue the medicine for three to four days.

- When the relief is complete and immediate after 4 doses, reduce the doses to three the next day and then reduce to two doses on third day and finally one dose a day on fourth day before finally stopping the medicine from fifth day.

- If there is relief by use of the first remedy, there is no need to take second medicine and follow the instructions for reducing the dosage as given in above paragraph.

- Similarly if the relief comes by use of second or third remedy, follow the above procedure.

IN ALPHABETICAL ORDER SOME OF THE DISEASES WITH THEIR REMEDIES

Name of the Disease/Disorder	Remedies		
	I	II	III

A

Name of the Disease/Disorder	I	II	III
Abdominal disorders	Nux-v.	Carbo-v.	Chin.
Abscess	Belladonna	Hep.	Merc.
Abuse of drugs, alcohol, tobacco	Nux-v.	Tabacum	Sul-ac.
Aching	Arn.	Rhus-t.	Chin.
Acidity	Calc.	Nux-v.	Sul-ac.

Acne (pimples on face of youths)	Asterias rub.	Kalium brom.	Calcarea phos.
Airsickness, vomiting	Borax (three doses a day before traveling by air)		
Alopecia (Falling of hair)	Lycopodium cla.	Acid phos.	Wiesbaden aq.
Anaemia	Calcarea phos.	China off.	Ferrum met.
Anus itching, due to worms	Cina	Teucrium	Spigelia ant.
Anus itching, burning, crawling	Sulphur	Ratanhia	Ignatia ama.
Anxiety	Aconite nap.	Ignatia ama.	Natrium mur.
Ankles- swelling	Apis/mel.	Stront-c.	Ledum pal.
Appetite, loss of	China off.	Nux-v.	Ferrum met.
Appetite increased or changed	Cina	Calcarea carb.	China off.
Aphthae (mouth ulcers or stomatitis)	Borax ven.	Merc. sol.	Acid nit.

B

Back-pain	Rhus tox.	Bryonia alb.	Antimonium tart.
Back pain, lifting from	Rhus tox.	Calcarea carb.	Graphites
Back pain with haemorrhoids	Aesculus hip.	Nux-v.	———
Back pain before menses	Kalium carb.	Pulsatilla	Lachesis mut.
Back pain during menses	Causticum	Kalium carb.	Pulsatilla
Back pain lower	Aesculus hip.	Cimicifuga rac.	Arnica mont.
Bad or foul breath	Merc sol.	Carbolicum acid	———
Barber's itch	Rhus tox.	Petroleum	Tellurium
Bed sores	Arnica mont.	Calendula off.	Acid fluor.
Bed-wetting	Cina	Sepia off.	Kreosotum

Bites	Apis (bees, insects)	Lyssinum (dogs)	Caladium (mosquito)
Belching	Antimonium crud.	Argentum nit.	Carbo veg.
Bleeding gums	Carbo veg.	Merc sol.	Arnica mont.
Bleeding piles	Acid nit.	Hamamelis	Ferrum phos.
Blood, loss of (haemorrhage)	China off.	Hamamelis	Phosphorus
Blood pressure high	Baryta mur.	Aurum met.	Lachesis mut.
Blood pressure, low	Cactus gran.	China off.	Carbo veg.
Blisters	Natrium mur. (around lips)	Cantharis (feet) Due to excess walks	Apis (insect bites)
Bone injuries	Symphytum	Arnica mont.	Ruta
Bone enlargement	Calcarea fluor.	Acid fluor.	Hecla lava
Bones pain	Eupatorium perf.	Ruta	Asafoetida
Breathlessness	Calcarea carb.	Arsenic alb.	Carbo veg.
Burns	Cantharis	Hepar sulphur	Kalium bich. (deep burns) (pus formed)
Burning of soles	Sulphur	Sanguinaria c.	Lycopodium cla.
Burning of palms	Sulphur	Petroleum	Phosphorus
Burning of chest	Carbo veg.	Sulphur	———
Burning of urine	Cantharis	Sulphur	Merc cor.
Burning of vagina	Carbo an.	Kreosotum	Sulphur

C

Car sickness, travel sickness	Cocculus ind.	Ignatia ama.	Petroleum
Changing or shifting pains	Kalium bich.	Pulsatilla	Lac can.

Children General Disorders/Awkward Behaviour

Weak, mentally or physically	Baryta carb.	Calcarea phos.	Kalium phos.
Is afraid of downward motions	Borax ven.	————	————
Irritable behaviour, quiet when carried	Chamomilla	————	————
Rachitic	Calcarea carb.	————	————
Complaints of pains in legs at night	Calcarea phos.		
Smells sour	Calcarea carb.	Hepar sulph.	Rheum
Desires things but refuses when given	Chamomilla	Bryonia	————
Pulls own hair	Belladonna	————	————
Very shy	Silicea ter.	————	————
Keeps hands moving on objects of the table	Kalium mur.	————	————
Shakes feet while sitting on chair	Lycopodium cla.	————	————
Tosses, kicks clothes off, restless sleep	Arsenicum alb.	————	————
Eats excessive salt	Natrium mur.	————	————
Eats excessive sweets	Argentum nit.	————	————
Chews cloth and raw food-rice	Alumina	————	————
Eats earth, lime, clay, chalk	Calcarea carb.	Alumina	Acid Nit.
Crying before urinating	Lycopodium cla.	Borax ven.	————
Crying during teething	Chamomilla	Calcarea phos.	————
Crying during teething, milk disagrees	Aethusa cyan.	————	————
Crying spells- withholding breathing, when crying	Ferrum met.	————	————
Colic, infantile	Allium cepa	Aloe	Chamomilla
Frightened in sleep	Lycopodium cla.	————	————
Late learning to talk	Natrium mur.*		
Late learning to walk	Calcarea carb.* *consult a doctor		
Constipation of infants	Alumina	Bryonia alb.	Magnesium carb.
Diarrhoea of children	Chamomilla	Podophyllum peli.	Calcarea carb
Diarrhoea of children during dentition	Calcarea carb.	Podophyllum peli	Chamomilla
Infants, nose block at night	Sambucus	————	————
Children pulling penis frequently	Merc sol.	Cantharis	————

Coryza (discharge from nose, eyes common cold)	Allium cepa	Arsenicum alb.	Natrium mur.
Coryza with irritating eyes	Euphrasia off.	———	———
Cold, dry weather increases it	Aconitum nap.	Calcarea carb.	Hepar sulp.
Cold, wet weather increases it	Rhus tox.	Calcarea carb.	Dulcamara
Cold, nose running during day and nose block at night		Nux-v.	
Calculus (stones) in kidneys	Berberis vulg.	Consult a doctor, if it fails	
Caries of teeth	Kreosotum	Merc sol.	Plantago maj.
Coccyx pain due to injury	Hypericum perf.	Graphites	———
Cervical spondylosis	Rhus tox.	Conium mac.	Acid phos.
Constipation, general	Nux-v.	Alumina	Bryonia alb.
Constipation, ineffectual urging	Lycopodium cla.	Nux-v.	Sulphur
Constipation alternating with diarrhoea	Antim crud.	Nux-v.	Chelidonium maj.
Constipation, before and during menses	Natrium mur.	Sepia off.	Silicea ter.
Constipation during pregnancy* (* Consult a doctor)	Alumina	Nux-v.	Sepia off.
Constipation, stool slips back	Silicea ter.	Thuja occ.	Sanicula aq.
Constipation of travelers	Platinum met.	Nux-v.	———
Constipation, no desire for days	Alumina	Bryonia alb.	Hydrastis
Corns	Antimonium crudum	Thuja occ.	Acidum nit.
Cough dry	Aconitum nap.	Belladonna	Ipecac
Cough, wet	Bryonia alb.	Belladonna	Antim tart.

Cough, eating aggravates	Bryonia alb.	Cocc-c	Kalium bi.
Cough of old people	Alumina	Antimonium tart.	Baryta carb.
Cough, urine escapes with	Causticum	Rumex	Pulsatilla
Cough, whooping	Carbo veg.	Ipecac	Drosera rot.
Cough, talking aggravate	Rumex cris.	Phosphorus	Drosera rot.
Cough with vomiting of food	Ipecac	Drosera rot.	Ferrum phos.
Coughing bring pain in head	Belladonna	Bryonia alb.	Capsicum
Chest pain with flatulence	Carbo veg.	———	———
Cramps, legs and calves	Ambra gris.	Cuprum met.	Magnesium phos.
Cracked lips, fingertips	Natrium mur.	Graphites	———
Cracking of joints	Causticum	Kalium bi.	Petroleum
Cramps	Colocynthis	Cuprum met.	Magnesium phos.

D

Dandruff	Calcarea carb.	Thuja occ.	Graphites
Dentition (teething)	Calcarea phos.	Ferrum phos.	———
Desire for salt	Causticum	Sepia off.	Conium mac.
Diarrhoea	Aconitum nap.	Aloe	China off.
Diarrhoea, hot weather	Podophyllum pel.	Antimonium crud.	Aloe
Diarrhoea, early morning	Sulphur	Podophyllum pel.	Natrium sulph.
Diarrhoea with flatus escaping	Argentum nit.	China off.	Aloe
Diarrhoea, offensive	Chamomilla	Podophyllum pel.	Arsenicum alb.
Diarrhoea with force like a shot	Podophyllum pel.	Croton tig.	———
Diarrhoea, sour stink	Calcarea carb.	Rheum	Hepar sulph.

Diarrhoea with rumbling	Aloe	Natrium sulph.	Acidum phos.
Diarrhoea with undigested particles	Calcarea carb.	China off.	Ferrum phos.
Drinks desired, very hot	Arsenicum alb.	Chelidonium maj.	———
Drinks desired, cold	Pulsatilla	Selenium met.	———
Drinks desired, very cold	Phosphorus	———	———
Drowsiness	Acidum phos.	Gelsemium sem.	———
Dryness of mouth	Bryonia alb.	Arsenicum alb.	———
Dryness of mouth, no thirst	Apis	Nux mos.	Pulsatilla
Dyspepsia (gastric symptoms)	Carbo veg.	China off.	Lycopodium cla.
Dysentery	Mercurius cor.	Ipecac	Ferrum phos.

E

Ear pain	Belladonna	Aconitum	Chamomilla
Ear discharge	Pulsatilla	Mercurius sol.	Hepar sulph.
Eating more (hungry)	Cina	Iodium	Sulphur
Eats well but looses weight	Abrotanum	Iodium	Natrium mur.
Ecchymosis (blueness of skin-'neel')	Arnica mont.	Ledum pal.	Acidum sulph.
Emotional, easily excited	Aconitum nap.	Arsenic alb.	Causticum
Eczema (general) see next chapter	Arsenicum alb.	Mercurius viv.	———
Epistaxis (Nose bleeding)	Bryonia alb.	Millefolium	Ipecac
Eructations	Argentum nit.	Carbo veg.	Sulphur
Eruptions in winter	Alumina	Petroleum	Psorinum
Examination fear	Anacardium occ.	Argentum nit.	Gelsemium sem.
Exostosis (bone enlargement)	Calcarea fluor.	Acidum fluor.	Hecla lava

Exposure to cold winds, all diseases	Aconitum nap.	Rhus tox.	————
Expulsion of foreign bodies	Silicea ter.	————	————
Extremities swollen	Apis	Mercurius sol.	Natrium mur.
Excessive sexual desire	Staphysgaria	Phosphorus	————
Eyes burning, tears bland	Allium cepa	Arsenicum alb.	————
Eyes red	Belladonna	Euphrasia off.	————
Eyes overstraining	Ruta	Natrium mur.	Senega
Eyes disorders, watering, red etc.	Euphrasia off.	————	————
Eyes lids glued together after sleep	Borax ven.	Pulsatilla	Argentum nit.
Eyes upper lids swelling	Kalium carb.	————	————
Eyes, swelling below	Apis	————	————
Eyes, dark rings around	China off.	Natrium carb.	Phosphorus

F

Fever, simple, exposure to cold	Aconitum nap	Bryonia alb.	Nux-v.

(Please see fever in details in the next chapter)

Formication (creeping sensation)	Aconitum nap.	Agaricus mus.	Natrium mur.
Flatulence (gas)	Carbo veg.	Pulsatilla	China off.
Facial blemishes	Berberis aqui.	Cimicifuga rac.	Sepia off.
Face, upper lip swelling	Hepar sulph.	Apis	Natrium mur.
Face, much oily, greasy	Natrium mur.	Thuja occ.	Psorinum
Face pain	Aconitum nap. (General)	Kalmia lat. (right)	Spigelia ant. (left)

Facial pain (right)	Kalmia lat.	Pulsatilla	Aconitum nap.
Facial pain (left)	Spigelia ant.	Colocynthis	———
Falling out of hair	Acidum phos.	Lycopodium cla.	Natrium mur.
Fastidiousness	Arsenicum alb.	Anacardium ori.	Nux-v.
Feet, sweat offensive	Silicea ter.	Calcarea carb.	———
Feet burning	Sanguinaria can	Chamomilla	Sulphur
Feet numbness	Arsenicum alb.	Natrium mur.	Acidum phos.
Feet heaviness	Alumina	Arsenicum alb.	Natrium mur.
Fidgety (Uneasiness of nerves, muscles of hands and feet)	Kalium brom.	Zincum met.	Phosphorus
Fissures and cracks	Graphites	Silicea ter.	———
Fingers, boring in nose by children	Cina	Sulphur	———
Fingers, crack	Calcarea carb.	Natrium mur.	Petroleum
Fistula	Calcarea carb.	Calcarea phos.	Silicea ter.
Forgetfulness of old persons	Lycopodium cla.	Acidum phos.	Baryta carb.
Fright, ailments from	Aconitum nap.	Ignatia am.	Opium
Fractures of bones	Arnica mont.	Symphytum off.	Ruta
Fungus growth, corns, warts	Thuja occ.	Causticum	Acidum Nit.
Forehead eruptions	Ledum pal.	Natrium mur.	Sepia off.
Forehead heaviness	Aconitum	Belladonna	Natrium mur.

G

Gallstone pain	Calcarea carb.	Berberis vulg.	China off.
Gastric problems	Carbo veg.	Pulsatilla	Calcarea carb.
Genitals burning, hot	Coffea cru.	Tarentula his.	———

Genitals, eruptions	Rhus tox.	Petroleum	Sulphur
Genitals, itching	Coffea cru.	Radium brom.	Natrium mur.
Genitals, offensive odour	Sarsaparilla	Sulphur	Thuja occ.
Giddiness (looking down)	Argentum nit.	Colocynthis	Silicea ter.
Giddiness (looking up)	Causticum	Pulsatilla	Kalium phos.
Glands, stony hard	Bromium	Conium mac.	Carbo an.
Glands swelling (general)	Rhus tox.	Mercurius sol.	Aurum met.
Grinding of teeth (sleep)	Cina	Belladonna	Calcarea carb.
Grief, effects of	Ignatia ama.	Natrium mur.	Causticum
Gripe of children (pain)	Chamomilla	Colocynthis	Magnesium phos.
Goitre	Calcarea carb.	Iodium	Spongia tos.
Gout, joints	Urtica urens-Q	Acidum Benz.	Ledum pal.
Greasy skin (oily)	Natrium mur.	Bryonia alb.	Causticum
Gums bleeding	Carbo veg.	Mercurius sol.	Acidum nit.
Gums, receding	Ammonium carb.	Mercurius sol.	Carbo veg.
Gums, painful boil and swelling	Borax ven.	Belladonna	Mercurius sol.

H

Haemorrhage	Please see blood, loss of in 'B'		
Haemorrhage after tooth extraction	Arnica mont.	Hamamelis vir.	Bovista lyc.
Haemorrhage, from uterus	Sabina	Hamamelis vir.	China off.
Haemorrhoids (piles), external	Aesculus hip.	Hamamelis vir.	Aloe
Haemorrhoids, internal	Nux vomica	Arsenic alb.	Sulphur
Haemorrhoids, blind	Aesculus hip.	Nux vomica	Sulphur
Haemorrhoids, bleeding	Acidum nit.	Hamamelis vir.	Hypericum per.
Haematuria (blood in urine)* (* Consult a doctor)	Sarsaparilla	Hepar sulph.	Lycopodium cla.

Haemoglobin, to raise	Ferrum phos. 3x	———	———
Hair loss of	Please see Alopecia in 'A'		
Hair falling in bunches, handfuls	Carbo veg.	Mezereum	Phosphorus
Hair falling after pregnancy and disease	Natrium mur.	Sepia off.	———
Hair on face on lips/chin of women* (*consult a doctor)	Thuja occ.	Oleum jec. 3x	———
Hair falling after parturition	Carbo veg.	Sulphur	Lycopodium cla.
Hair oily and greasy	Bryonia alb.	Mercurius sol.	Acidum phos.
Hair dry	Calcarea carb.	Thuja occ.	Sulphur
Hard bed, lying on sensation	Arnica mont.	Baptisia tin.	Pyrogenium
Headache, frontal	Aconitum nap.	Belladonna	Byronia alb.
Headache, frontal extending to eyes, Nose or face	Agaricus mus.	Byronia alb.	Aloe
Headache, frontal extending to back of head, neck and spine	Byronia alb.	Gelsemium sem.	Lac def.
Headache, back of head	Bryonia alb.	Cimicifuga rac.	Nux vomica
Headache from back of head to Eyes and forehead	Gelsemium sem.	Sanguinaria can.	Silicea ter.
Headache left sided	Spigelia ant.	Colocynthis	Lachesis mut.
Headache, right-sided	Belladonna	Sanguinaria can.	Calcarea carb.
Headache of school -girls	Calcarea phos.	Natrium mur.	———
Headache periodical	Sanguinaria can.	———	———
Headache goes from left to right	Lachesis mut.	———	———
Headache goes from right to left	Belladonna	———	———
Head-lice* (*Externally, use lotion	Natrium mur.	Carbolicum acid.	Psorinum

of sabadilla at night and wash in the morning. Comb hair with lice-comb duly dipped in lukewarm water after each combing- stroke. Repeated strokes each day help. Special lice combs are available in the market)

Head problems, late effect of injuries	Arnica mont.	Natrium sulph.	Natrium mur.
Healing is poor in ulcers, boils	Hepar sulph.	Mercurius sol.	Silicea ter.
Heat, burning sensation	Arsenicum alb.	Sanguinaria can.	Sulphur
Heart -burn	Please see gastric problems under 'G'		
Heaviness of stomach after eating	China off.	Nux vomica	Pulsatilla
Heaviness of abdomen, load	Lycopodium cla.	Aloe	Graphites
Heaviness of bladder	Lycopodium cla.	Natrium mur.	Sepia
Heaviness of uterus	China off.	Sepia	———
Heels pain	Pulsatilla	Causticum	Cyclamen
Hernia (*consult a doctor)	Lycopodium cla.*	Nux vomica	Acidum nit.
Hiccoughs	Magnesium phos. 12x	Nux vomica	Ignatia am.
Hips, painful	Arnica mont.	Phytolacca dec.	Ruta
Hoarseness	Causticum	Arum trip.	Sulphur
Home sickness	Ignatia ama.	Bryonia alb.	Acidum phos.
Hunger, more (Also see appetite) With loss of flesh	Iodum	Abrotanum	Natrium mur.
Hypertension and hypotension	Please see blood pressure in 'B'		
Hydrocele* (consult a doctor)	Rhododendron	Graphites	Pulsatilla

I

Inability to think	Natrium sulph.	Natrium carb.	Nux mos.
Inactive lethargic	Nux mos.	Acidum phos.	Gelsemium sem.
Incontinence of urine or stool	Causticum	Acidum phos.	Kreosoteum
Indifferent to others (apathy)	Acidum phos.	Sepia	Ambra gris. (to all things)
Indigestion* (* see dyspepsia under 'D')	Pulsatilla	Nux vomica	Aethusa (When over-fed)
Impotency	Acidum phos.	Selenium met.	Staphysagria
Impotency due to masturbation	Staphysagria	Agnus castus	Lycopodium cla.
Inflammation of eye-lids	Graphites	Mezereum	Argentum nit.
Influenza	Eupatorium perf.	Rhus tox.	Gelsemium sem.
Injury to eyes	Symphytum off.	———	———
Injury to eye-ball	Arnica mont.	Ledum pal.	Symphytum off.
Injury due to fracture	Symphytum	Arnica mont.	Calcarea phos.
Injury to head	Arnica mont.	Natrium sulph.	———
Injury, sprains, strains	Rhus tox.	Calcarea carb.	Nux vomica
Insects bite	Apis mel.	Ledum pal.	Arsenicum alb.
Insomnia, sleeplessness	Aconitum nap.	Ignatia am.	Coffea crud.
Insult, bad effects of	Anacardium ori.	Ignatia am.	Colocynthis
Involuntary sighing	Ignatia am.	Calcarea phos.	Lachesis mut.
Involuntary stool in children	Aloe	———	———
Itching on undressing	Rumex cris.	Natrium sulph.	Oleander
Itching, Scratches till it bleeds	Mezereum	Arsenicum alb.	Psorinum
Itching without eruptions	Dolichos prur	Arsenicum alb.	Mezereum
Itching, burning after	Rhus tox.	Petroleum	Sulphur
Itching, anus	Cina	Aloe	Sulphur

J

Jaundice	Chelidonium maj.	Lycopodium cla.	Nux vomica
Jaundice, liver painful	China off.	Podophyllum pel.	Sepia off.
Jaws swelling	Hecla lava	Kreosotum	Acidum nit.
Joints,cracking	Causticum	Ginseng quin.	Aconitum nap.
Joints pain	Eupatorium perf.	Argentum met.	Symphytum off.
Joy, excessive, ill effects, insomnia	Coffea	———	———

K

Keloids	Acidum fluo.	Silicea ter.	Thuja occ.
Kidney disorders*	Berberis vul.	Apis mel.	Terebinthina ch.
Kidney stone* (*Consult a doctor)	Berberis vul.	Calcarea carb.	Ocimum can.
Knees pain, simple	Berberis vul.	Dioscorea vil.	Rhus tox.
Knees pain, rheumatic	Acidum Ben.	Causticum	Phytolacca dec.
Knees, synovitis (lack of bone lubricant)	Apis mel.	Sulphur	Bryonia alb.
Knees, swelling	Apis mel.	Ledum pal.	Acidum nit.

L

Lactation (Breast milk) late coming and suppressed later	Aconitum nap.	Asafoetida	Calcarea carb.
Lactation, absence of milk	Millefolium	———	———
Lactation, for terminating	Lac can.	Pulsatilla	———
Laryngitis	Aconitum nap.	Spongia tos.	Kalium bi.

Lassitude (weariness)	Sepia off.	Acidum phos.	Ferrum phos.
Laughing causing more of disease	Borax ven.	Stannum met.	Phosphorus
Laughing on matters (triffles) that are insignificant	Cannabis indi.	Hyoscyamus nig.	———
Lethargic	Nux mos.	Gelsemium sem.	———
Leucorrhoea	Calcarea carb.	Sepia off.	Borax ven.
Lentigo (freckles) brown	Calcarea carb.	Pulsatilla	Sulphur
Lice in head	See 'Head'		
Lifting weight, causing pain, strains	Arnica mont.	Rhus tox.	———
Lips crack	Natrium mur.	Sepia off.	Psorinum
Liver disorders, general	Chelidonium maj.	Lycopodium cla.	China off.
Liver enlarged	Natrium sulph.	Lycopodium cla.	———
Loquacity (talking too much)	Lachesis mut.	Stramonium	Hyoscyamus nig.
Lumbar region pain	See Back pains under 'B'		
Lump feeling in throat	Asafoetida	Ignatia ama.	———
Lying down frequently, desire	Gelsemium sem.	Nux vomica	Silicea ter.
Lying down causes aggravaion	Rhus tox.	Pulsatilla nig.	Natrium sulph.
Lying down causes amelioration	Nux vomica	Bryonia alb.	———
Lying right side cause aggravation	Rhus tox.	Magnesium mur.	Stannum met.
Lying left side cause aggravation	Pulsatilla nig.	Spigelia ant.	Kalium carb.
Lying right side cause amelioration	Natrium mur.	Sulphur	———
Lying left side cause amelioration	Ignatia ama.	Stannum met.	———
Lying painful side cause amelioration	Bryonia alb.	Pulsatilla nig.	Calcarea carb.

M

Masturbation habit, ill effects	Acidum phos.	Staphysagria	———
Measles	Pulsatilla nig.	Arsenic alb.	Euphrasia off.
Menopause	Lachesis mut.	———	———
Menstruation disturbances, general* (* See next chapter for detailed symptoms)	Pulsatilla nig.	Sepia off.	———
Menses, complaints before and after	Natrium mur.	———	———
Menses, complaints after	Borax ven.	Graphites	———
Menses, complaints during	Pulsatilla nig.	Graphites	———
Menses, complaints before	Pulsatilla nig.	Calcarea carb.	Sulphur
Menses, complaints when lying down	Kreosotum	Magnesium carb.	———
Mental tiredness	Kalium phos.	Nux vomica	Gelsemium sem.
Mental development slow* (Consult a doctor, a long process of healing)	Baryta carb.	Natrium mur.	Calcarea carb.
Milk, intolerance by children (not digested)	Aethusa cyan.	Magnesium carb.	Natrium carb.
Mouth, offensive odour, sleeping	Mercurius sol.	Aethusa cyan.	Carbo veg.
Mouth ulcers, general	Borax ven.	Acidum nit.	Mercurius sol.
Mouth bitter, bad taste	Pulsatilla nig.	Mercurius sol.	———
Mouth blisters, corners	Natrium mur.	Pulsatilla nig.	Mercurius sol.
Mouth dryness but with thirst	Bryonia alb.	———	———
Mumps	Belladonna	Mercurius iod.	Phytolacca dec.
Muscles, sprains, strains	Arnica mont.	Rhus tox.	Causticum

N

Nails, ingrowing	Silicea ter.	Graphites	Magnesium phos.

Nails cracked	Natrium mur.	Antimonium crud.	Silicea ter.
Nails, grow quickly	Acidum fluor.	———	———
Nails, do not grow	Antimonium crud.	———	———
Nails, white spots	Silicea ter.	———	———
Nails biting	Natrium mur.	Arum trip.	———
Nausea	Ipecac	Arsenicum alb.	Nux vomica
Nausea in pregnancy	Sepia off.	———	———
Naval bleeding, infants	Abrotanum	Nux mos.	———
Neck pain	Cimicifuga rac.	Rhus tox.	Bryonia alb.
Neck stiff	Aconitum nap.	Belladonna	Causticum
Neuralgia (pain) of face, left	Spigelia ant.	———	———
Neuralgia, face right side	Aconitum nap.	Pulsatilla nig.	Kalmia lat.
Neuralgia anywhere with numbness	Chamomilla	———	———
Nerves painful	Aconitum nap.	Belladonna	Magnesium phos.
Nose bleeding, not knowing cause	Belladonna	Ferrum phos.	———
Nose bleeding in the morning	Ambra gris.	———	———
Nose bleeding when washing face	Ammonium carb.	———	———
Nose blocking on sleeping	Sambucus nig.	Lycopodium cla.	———
Nose blocking when going out	Hepar sulphur	———	———
Nose boring by children till it bleeds	Arum trip.	———	———
Nose boring by children, frequent	Cina	———	———
Nose, polypi	Lemna minor	———	———
Nose running	Allium cepa	Arsenicum alb.	Euphrasia off.
Numbness, general	Natrium mur.	Aconitum nap.	Rhus tox.

Numbness of feet, hands or soles	Alumina	———	———
Numbness of head	Asafoetida	Kalium phos.	———
Numbness, lying on limbs	Carbo veg.	Pulsatilla nig.	Rhus tox.

O

Obesity	Fucuc ves. Q	Calcarea carb.	Phytolacca berry
Odour offensive from body	Mercurius sol.	Psorinum	———
Odour, intolerance for strong odours	Nux vomica	———	———
Odour, offensive feet-sweats	Calcarea carb.	Silicea ter.	———
Oedema, below eyes	Apis mel.	———	———
Oedema, upper lids, eyes	Kalium carb.	———	———
Oedema, general	Apis mel.	Arsenicum alb.	Colchicum
Offended easily	Staphysagria	Ignatia ama.	Nux vomica
Old age disorders, general (senility, sexual excesses, trembling, weakness etc.)	Ambra gris.	Baryta carb.	Lycopodium cla.
Operation, after effects	Rhus tox.	Hypericum per.	Cimicifuga rac.
Orchitis, inflammation of testicles	Clematis erecta	Spongia tos.	Mercurius cor.
Otorrhoea, discharge from ears	Pulsatilla nig.	Hepar sulphur	Mercurius sol.
Ovary pain	Colocynthis	Podophyllum pel.	Lachesis mut.
Over lifting, pains thereof	Rhus tox.	———	———
Ozeana, offensive nasal discharge	Asafoetida	Mercurius cor.	Calcarea carb.

P

Pains, body Worse during rest	Rhus tox.	Kalium carb.	Magnesium phos.

Pains deep in bones	Aurum met.	Asafoetida	Eupatorium perf.
Pain in long bones	Eupatorium perf.	Staphysagria	Mezereum
Pains in damp weather	Rhus tox.	Dulcamara	Mercurius sol.
Pains, dull type	China off.	Nux vomica	Ignatia ama.
Pains, burning type	Apis mel.	Arsenicum alb.	Sulphur
Pains bursting type	Aconitum nap.	Bryonia	Capsicum an.
Pains squeezing type	Cactus gran.	Acidum nit.	Sulphur
Pains stitching type	Bryonia alb.	Natrium sulph.	Kalium carb.
Pains in scapulae, (shoulders)	Chelidonium maj.	Sanguinaria can.	Ferrum met.
Pains, cramps type	Cuprum met.	Colocynthis	Pulsatilla nig.
Pains during night only	Aurum met.	Asafoetida	Mercurius sol.
Pains with periodicity (Definite time interval)	Sanguinaria can.	Arsenicum alb.	China off.
Pains wandering	Pulsatilla nig.	Kalium bi.	Kalmia lat.
Pains suddenly come, suddenly go	Belladonna	Kalium bi.	Kalium carb.
Palpitations at night	Calcarea carb.	Cannabis indica	Lachesis mut.
Perspiration, excessive	Acidum phos.	Rhus glabra	Thuja occ.
Pharyngitis	Belladona	Kalium bi.	Mercurius sol.
Piles	Please see haemorrhoids in 'H'		
Pimples, general (please see acne in 'A')	Belladonna	Carbo veg.	Kalium brom.
Plugging of nails, sensation	Ignatia am.	Thuja occ.	Anacardium ori.
Polyp, nasal	Sanguinaria nit.	Calcarea carb.	Teucrium mar.
Polyuria	Argentum nit.	Calcarea fluor.	Acid. phos.
Prolapse of rectum	Sepia off.	Ruta gra.	Podophyllum pel.
Prolapse of uterus	Sepia off.	Natrium mur.	Belladonna
Prostatitis* (* Consult a doctor)	Sabal ser. Q	Conium mac.	Ferrum pic.

Ptyalism (excessive saliva)	Mercurius sol.	Kalium mur.	Syph. 200, one dose
Puffiness of face	Apis mel.	Arsenicum alb.	Calcarea carb.
Pus forming, boils	Mercurius sol. (About to form)	Hepar sulphur (Already formed)	Hepar sulphur 200 (To abort, one dose)
Pruritis (itching)	Rhus tox.	Rumex cris.	Sulphur
Pyrrhoea, bad smell from mouth	Merc cor.	Kalium carb.	Carbo veg. (When bleeding too)

R

Rash, mosquito bite	Dulcamara	———	———
Rash, children	Aconitum nap.	Bryonia alb.	———
Restlessness	Aconitum nap.	Arsenicum alb.	Rhus tox.
Ringworm	Sepia off.	Arsenicum alb.	Bacillinum-1M (one dose)
Rectum, fullness	Aesculus hip.	Acidum nit.	Sulphur
Rectum, burning	Arsenicum alb.	Capsicum an.	Sulphur
Rectum, continuous pain	Acidum nit.	Aesculus hip.	Phytolacca dec.
Rhinitis, first stage	Aconitum nap.	Arsenicum alb.	Gelsemium sem.
Ribs pain	Aconitum nap.	Wyethia hel.	Argentum nit.

S

Sad, feeling of	Ignatia ama.	Natrium mur.	Aurum met.
Saliva, more	Mercurius sol.	Allium sativa	Ammonium carb.
Sciatica, general	Colocynthis	Rhus tox.	Gnaphalium poly.
Scabies	Calcarea sulph. (Dry or wet)	Graphites (wet)	Hepar sulphur

Seasickness	Nux vomica	Cocculus ind.	Petroleum
*Sexual desire, lost or diminished	Lycopodium cla.	Staphysagria	———
Sexual desire excessive (Male, better consult a doctor)	Cantharis ves. (painful erection)	Acidum fluor.	Acidum phos.
Skin affections, eczema wet	Graphites	———	———
Skin affections, Itching and burning	Sulphur	———	———
Skin sensitive to touch and cold	Hepar sulphur	———	———
Sensation of fullness (stomach)	Lycopodium cla.	Aesculus hip.	China off.
Sensation of emptiness (stomach)	Sepia off.	Coccus cac.	———
Sinusitis	Kalium bich.	Silicea ter.	Sanguinaria can.
Sleepiness	Cimex lec.	Cyclamen Euro.	———
Smell of food intolerable	Colchicum	Sepia off.	Arsenicum alb.
Sneezing, persistent	Sabadilla	Sanguinaria can.	Cyclamen
Sneezing without coryza (common cold)	Calcarea carb.	Mercurius sol.	Acidum nit.
Sneezing morning	Kalium bi.	Allium cepa	Ammonium carb.
Sneezing violent	Agaricus mus.	Cyclamen Euro.	———
Snoring	Lemna minor	Hippozaeninum	Sanguinaria nit.
Sore throat	Belladonna	Mercurius sol.	Hepar sulphur
Soreness	Rhus tox.	Arnica mont.	Ruta grav.
Sourness	Calcarea carb.	———	———
Spondylitis, left sided	Ferrum phos.	Rhus tox.	Causticum
Spondylitis, right sided (Please see cervical under 'C' also)	Chelidonium maj.	Natrium mur.	Carbo an.

Spots, pain in small spots	Kalium bi.	Lachesis mut.	———
Spots, yellow and brown on face	Sepia off.	Sulphur	———
Stammering	Bovista Lyc.	Stramonium	———
Standing uncomfortable	Sulphur	———	———
Sticky discharges, cough, stool etc.	Kalium bi.	Graphites	———
Stiffness of body parts	Rhus tox.	Bryonia alb.	———
Stinging, sensation	Silicea ter.	Apis mel.	———
Stomach disorders, indigestion	Nux vomica	Carbo veg.	Lycopodium cla.
Stomach, burning	Arsenicum alb.	Sepia off.	Sulphur
Stomach heaviness after eating (Also see 'sensation' above)	Lycopodium cla.	Kalium bich.	Hepar sulphur
Stomatitis	Please see mouth ulcers in 'M'		
Stool, frequent, desire ineffectual	Nux vomica	Sepia off.	Aloe
Stool, dry, hard, burnt	Bryonia alb.	———	———
Stool, slips back	Silicea ter.	Thuja occ.	Sanicula aq.
Stool with mucus, knotty, large	Graphites	———	———
Stool, no desire for days	Alumina	Bryonia alb.	Hydrastis Q
Stool passes only when standing	Causticum	———	———
Styes, eyes	Staphysagria	Thuja occ.	Silicea ter.
Sun-stroke	Glonoinum	Natrium carb.	Natrium mur.
Sweating, head	Calcarea carb.	———	———
Sweating on uncovered parts	Thuja occ.	———	———
Sweat offensive, foot or axilla	Rhus tox.	Sulphur	Silicea ter.
Sweat, missing- no sweating	Alumina	———	———

Swelling	Please see oedema in 'O'		
Swelling with pain	Apis mel.	Pulsatilla nig.	Acid. Nit.
Synovitis (Inflammation of joints having lubricating fluid)	Bryonia alb.	Calcarea fluor.	Apis mel.

T

Taste, bitter	Natrium mur.	Pulsatilla nig.	———
Taste, everything salty	Belladonna	———	———
Tasteless, tongue coated white	Antimonium Crud.	Natrium mur.	Magnesium carb.
Taste sour	Nux vomica	Calcarea carb.	Lycopodium cla.
Teeth bleeding after extraction	Arnica mont.	Staphysagria	Phosphorus
Teeth grinding	Cina	Belladonna	———
Teething troubles, children	Calcarea phos.	———	———
Thirst less, dry mouth	Pulsatilla nig.	Aethusa cyan. (Complete absence)	Apis mel.
Thirst more but of little quantity	Arsenicum alb.	———	———
Thirst unquenchable	Natrium mur.	Bryonia alb.	———
Throat sore	Please see sore throat under 'S'		
Thumb sucking (consult a doctor)	Calcarea phos.	Natrium mur.	Silicea ter.
Tongue mapped and cracked	Natrium mur.	Arum trip.	Rhus ven.
Tongue swelling with bad odour	Mercurius sol.	———	———
Tonsils red and inflamed	Belladonna	Mercurius sol.	Hepar sulphur
Tonsils, enlarged	Baryta carb.	Calcarea fluor.	Mercurius iod. rub.
Toothache	Mercurius sol.	Arsenicum alb.	Chamomilla
Twitching	Agaricus mus.	Ignatia ama.	Zincum met.

U

Ulcers with itching	Sulphur	———	———
Ulcers not healing quickly	Silicea ter.	———	———
Unrefreshing sleep	Nux vomica	———	———
Urination while, child cries	Borax ven.	———	———
Urine escapes involuntary	Causticum	Natrium mur.	———
Urine milky in children	Cina	Acidum phos.	———
Urine retention in children	Aconitum nap.	———	———
Urine urge more in newly weds	Staphysagria	———	———
Urticaria	Apis mel.	Urtica urens Q	Rhus tox.

V

Vaccination, ill effects	Thuja occ.	Silicea ter.	———
Varicose veins, legs	Aesculus hip.	Pulsatilla nig.	Acidum fluor.
Vertigo	Please see next chapter		
Voice loss, sudden of singers, speakers (See under hoarseness under 'H')	Arum trip.	Rhus tox.	Phosphorus
Vomiting	Ipecac (general)	Aethusa cyan. (After milk in infants)	Mercurius sol.
Vomiting in pregnancy	Sepia off.	———	———

W

Wakes up, frightened, suffocated	Spongia tos.	Sambucus nig.	———
Wandering pains	Pulsatilla nig.	Kalium bich.	Lac can.

Warts	Thuja occi.	Acidum nit.	Causticum
Wasp bite	Cantharis ves.	———	———
Watering from eyes	Euphrasia off.	———	———
Weakness feeling, general	China off.	Ferrum phos.	Acidum phos.
Weakness of old age	Ambra gris.	———	———
Weak memory	Anacardium ori.	Kalium phos.	———
Weak digestion after fever	Carbo veg.	Sepia off.	———
Weeps more	Ignatia ama.	Natrium mur.	Pulsatilla nig.
Weight loss though eats well	Iodum	Natrium mur.	Abrotanum
Worms	Cina	Teucrium mar.	———
Wrists cramps	Actaea spicata	Rhododendron	———
Writer's cramps	Gelsemium sem.	Argentum met.	Magnesium phos.

Y

Yawning, frequent	Aconitum nap. (more after lying)	Nux vomica (more after eating)	Ignatia ama.

———————

Part –III

According to Symptoms Single Remedy Prescription

Except in two or three cases of toothache and boils where alternating remedies are given to give quickest relief.

RULES OF TAKING MEDICINES

- Take the medicine in the potency and frequency shown.

- Where no potency is given, consider the medicine having 30th potency.

- Take a single dose of 4 pills in the morning on empty stomach, if not otherwise mentioned against the remedy.

- For children above 4 years, the dose is 4 pills.

- For children from 2 to 4 years, the dose is of 3 pills.

- For infants below 2 years, the dose is of 1 pill.

- Wait for 3 days for the results, if no other remarks are given against the medicines.

- In case of partial relief, reduce the dose to one a day and wait for another 3 days.

- If complete relief comes, no repetition of dose is needed after three days.

- If no relief comes after a week, consult a doctor.

Acne

KNOW ABOUT ACNE ?

ACNE NOTIFIES pimples on the face, neck, shoulders or back. It is eruption of pustular, follicular or papular type in which sebaceous glands of the (oil producing) skin is involved. The reason behind acne is sensitiveness to normal level of sex hormones. This over-sensitiveness produces high level of sebum (oily secretions). Its effect comes with onset of adolescence. Teenagers are the victims of this disorder and boys are more prone to it than girls. Acne brings in a sort of inferiority complex or distress to the sufferer but does not cause any serious harm to health.

First Step Treatment

- A lot of 'Salad' with meals, more of milk, curd and butter do help erase acne.

- Washing the face with oil-free soap after returning to home from outside is helpful.

- Avoid more of perspiration by avoiding hot spicy food, junk food and cold drinks.

- Take eatables having more of vitamin A (milk, butter, eggs etc. No excessive intake of these items).

Note : Medicines to be taken three times a day for seven days when no other directive is written against medicine.

- At puberty, acne with itching: *Asterias rubens*.

- When Asterias rub. fails, and eruptions are pustular: *Kalium bromatum*.

- Pimples with constipation, pimples worse from bath: *Magnesia muriaticum*.

- Acne on nose: *Causticum.*

- Acne on forehead: *Ledum palustre.*

- Pimples are hard: *Agaricus muscarius.*

- Pimples are moist, digestion slow, flatulence: *Carbo vegetabilis.*

- Rosy pimples, pale skin and chilly feeling: *Silicea terra.*

- During menses acne is more and it is worse eating sugar, fats, meat, heavy meals, tea and coffee etc.: *Psorinum* 200 weekly one dose

- Young girls with menstrual disorders and debility *Calcarea phosphorica.*

Abdomen-Pains
KNOW ABOUT ABDOMINAL PAIN ?

ABDOMINAL PAIN is related to digestive system and reasons are many including infection, ulcers, appendicitis, constipation, gallstones etc. In reasons other than digestion, it may be a urinary tract infection, problems with kidneys, muscles straining or hernia. If the pains are persistent and continue for longer periods, make recurrence and are accompanied by fever, diarrhoea, vomiting and urinary troubles, it is better to consult a homoeopath. If the pains are of digestive relations, following medicines can be tried. In the case of digestive problem pains, it is better to eat light meals, high fibre diet and avoid eating fatty, rich, oily and spicy food. Take measures to avoid constipation. Drink lot of water and a glass of milk at bedtime. Try to be calm and free of stress.

First Step Treatment

- Smear some mustard oil on palms, massage the

abdomen in a circular direction very gently and slowly
till the patient feels comfortable.

- A hot compress can be given through a hot water bottle,
  on the painful area.

- Put two drops of *Bell-adonna* 200 dilution in half cup
  of water and give it to the patient every five minutes
  until the pain stops.

Note : Take the medicines three times a day for three days where no
other direction is mentioned. Take the potency as 30, if not
mentioned against the medicine.

Medicines

□ Burning pains relieved by warm applications, digestive
troubles after decayed food, non-vegetarian food, and
alcohol, chewing tobacco. Pains with restlessness and
thirst for little water at a time, feeling of chilliness:
Arsenic album for five days.

□ Pain on empty stomach: *Anacardium occidentale.*

□ Pain after eating: *Abies nigra.*

□ Pain with ineffectual desire for stool, sits for stool but
passes small stool at a time, distension after two hours
of taking meals: *Nux vomica* for 5 days.

□ Violent pain. It is better by hard pressure and bending
double: *Colocynthis.*

□ Stitching pains worse movement and especially if it is
before menses: *Kali carbonica* for one day only.

□ Pain is more after taking fatty, rich food. There is
discharge of flatus: *Pulsatilla nigricans* for five
days.

□ Pain abdomen radiating to other parts of the body and
obstinate constipation: *Plumbum metallicum.*

- Pain is more in upper abdomen. The stools are hard and constipated: *Graphites.*

- In front abdomen, pain is more. Tongue is clean but there is vomiting or nausea: *Ipecacuanha.*

- Pain shifting from abdomen to distant parts like fingers and toes. Pain better bending backwards and stretching the body: *Dioscorea.*

- Pain after operation of abdomen: *Staphysagria* for five days.

- Pain after over-eating, over-drinking alcohol and due to sedentary habits: *Nux vomica* for five days.

- Pain with acidity and burning. There is desire for fresh air and fanning: *Carbo vegetabilis* for five days.

- If pain is due to worms, patient bores his nose, grinds teeth in sleep, has itching in anus and has more of saliva: *Cina* for six days.

- Pain of pregnant women and pains are more after anger: *Chamomilla.*

Allergic to and
Food Aggravations
KNOW ABOUT ALLERGY ?

ALLERGY IS being sensitive to some food, drinks, climate, medicines etc. Allergy is triggered by exposure to an allergy causing substance/condition. The best way is to avoid the allergic substances and exposures but this is hardly possible till the actual cause of allergy is known. People cannot avoid dust and pollution in daily life of a polluted city. The alternative remains with making our immune system of body stronger so that resistence of the body to fight diseases is increased. Homoeopathy is capable of doing this.

First Step Treatment

- If it is dust allergy, avoid it by wrapping a piece of cloth on mouth and nose. The intensity of allergy will be less.

- There is no other measure to avoid allergies until the allergen is known. If one knows that taking onions cause coryza, he should stop taking it and take homoeopathic medicines so that he can restart taking onions.

Medicines

- Bread, acidic food: *Natrium muriaticum 200,* one dose early in the morning on empty stomach weekly for three weeks.

- Butter: *Pulsatilla nigricans 200* in the same as given above.

- Beer: *Kalium bichromicum 200* in the same manner as given above.

- Milk: *Magnesia carbonica 30,* three times a day for seven days.

- Cold milk: *Kalium iodatum 200,* one dose weekly on empty stomach for three weeks.

- Salted butter, aspirin, bad eggs, bad liquor, and poultry items: *Carbo vegetabilis 200* in the same manner as given above.

- Antibiotic medicines: *Sulphur 200,* one dose on empty stomach in morning in the same manner as given above.

- Coffee: *Nux vomica 200,* one dose in the same manner as given above.

- Heat: *Apis 30*, two times a day for seven days.

- Ice: *Arsenicum album 200*, weekly one dose at bed time, total three doses in three weeks.

- Cold drinks, fruits, over-ripe or rotten fruit and food: *Arsenicum album 200* in the same manner as above.

- Cold food: *Arsenicum album 200*, in the same manner as above.

- Hot food: *Bryonia alba* 200 in the same manner as above.

- Dampness: *Dulcamara 30*, three times a day for seven days.

- Sugar: *Argentum nitricum 200* weekly one dose at night for three weeks (three doses).

- Rice: *Tellurium 200*, in the same manner as above.

- Cabbage: *Petroleum 200* in the same manner as above.

- Decayed vegetables: *Carbo animalis 200* in the same manner as above.

- Pastry, ice cream, mixed variety food: *Pulsatilla nigricans 200* in the same manner as above.

- Lemons: *Selenium metallicum 200* in the same manner as above.

- Melons: *Zingiber officinale 30*, two doses a day for seven days.

- Pickles, sour food, acids: *Lachesis mutus 200*, weekly one dose for three weeks.

- Strawberries: *Oxalicum acidum 200* in the same manner as above.

- Onions: *Thuja occidentalis 200* in the same manner as above.

- Potatoes: *Alumina 200*, in the same manner as above.

- Meat: *Arsenicum album 200* in the same manner as above.

- Ornaments: *Argentum nitricum 200* in the same manner as above.

- Hair dye: *Sulphur 200*, on empty stomach in the same manner as above.

- Wheat flour, new or old: *Psorinum 200* in the same manner as above.

Appetite, Loss of or (Anorexia)

KNOW ABOUT LOSS OF APPETITE ?

AT TIMES when the body-system is not working properly, one does not feel like eating although pleasure of eating is irresistable. Loss of appetite may be due to fever, indigestion, and intake of excessive alcohol, pregnancy, sickness or reasons relating to worries. Let the reason may be anything but it is a temporary phase and once the food- style, the tensions of life and the sickness is removed, the appetite returns to normal. No harm is done to the body for want of appetite but if there is continuous loss of appetite, it may be serious. It could relate to cancer, hepatitis, hypertension, infections and rheumatoid arthritis etc. In continuous loss of appetite when ordinary medicines are not working, doctor should be consulted.

First Step Treatment

- If you have habit of taking too much tea or coffee, reduce their intake.

- Try regular exercise or walking for long distance every day.

- If you are a smoker or eat tobacco, stop it or cut down the quota.

- If you have extensive worries of family affairs or business etc., try to avoid them by finding an early solution. Expose your problems to nears and dears. This will relieve you of your tensions to some extent.

- If you take alcohol, reduce its quantity.

- If you have been taking three 'chapatis' in one meal and think that taking less than three is loss of appetite, you are wrong. Taking even one 'chapati' is sufficient but make the intake of food frequent, little at a time according to your existing little appetite. Eat small but regular meals in time.

- Taking some sour or bitter preparation like pickles, tomato curry, vegetable soup, 'Rasam' or fried ginger before meals will increase your appetite.

Medicines

- Hungry without appetite: *China officinalis 200*, one dose weekly for two weeks.

- Hungry without appetite and vomiting after eating: *Ferrum metallicum 30*, three times a day for seven days.

- Appetite lost but likes salt in every thing taken: *Natrium muriaticum 200*, one dose weekly for three weeks (total three doses).

- Pain in liver region and loss of appetite: *Chelidonium majus 200* in the same above manner.

- Loss of appetite in the morning but desires food in afternoon and night: *Abies nigra 200* in the same above manner.

- No appetite due to indigestion, taste in the mouth bitter and tongue coated: *Nux vomica 200* at bedtime one dose, three doses in three weeks.

- The stomach feels full after taking little food: *Lycopodium clavatum 200* only one dose in the morning. Wait for one week. If the complaint persists, take another dose. No more repetitions.

- Desire for variety of acidic and indigestible food but no desire for ordinary food: *Ignatia amara 200*, one dose at bedtime weekly for two weeks.

- Head remedy and general tonic for loss of appetite when no specific reason of loss of appetite is known: *Alfalfa-Q*, ten drops in half cup of water twice daily before meals for 10 days.

Arthritis, Gout, Rheumatism, Joint Pains
KNOW ABOUT ARTHRITIS ETC. ?

THERE ARE many types of the disease like osteoarthritis, rheumatoid arthritis, infective arthritis and gout etc. For a layman, they have a common symptom of pain in joints, stiffness and limited movement. Arthritis is a chronic condition of disease and it is included here in very brief way so that first hand treatment can be given. There will be relief from the pains temporarily after taking the medicines as per symptoms of the body, but it will be to the benefit of the patient to consult a homoeopath for proper treatment.

First Step Treatment : None

Medicines

- Joints of fingers, hands and feet painful, aggravation during menses or at the beginning of menopause: *Caulophyllum thalictroides-Q*, 10 drops in half cup of water, three times a day for seven days.

- Complaints worse during rest and exposure to cold, better by movements: *Rhus toxicodendron 200*, one dose in the morning empty stomach. Wait for three days. If pains are less, take the same medicine after four days, one dose and then weekly one dose for four weeks. In case of no improvement after first three days, consult the Homoeopath or try next medicine, if it has symptoms as stated below.

- When Rhus toxicodendron fails to work, pain worse in cold, better by movement: *Calcarea carbonica 200* in the same manner as above.

- Pain of joints with swelling and pains increase with movement: *Bryonia alba 200* in the same manner as above.

- Long bones pains: *Causticum 200* in the same manner as above.

- Long bones pain due to injury or with eye pain symptoms: *Ruta graveolens*, three times a day for seven days.

- Long bones pain, hip joint pain, pain better by motion: *Acidum phosphoricum 200* as mentioned against Rhus tox.

- Pain of large muscles, pain more at night, in wet weather: *Cimicifuga racemose 200*, two times a day for three days.

- Pain traveling downwards affecting large part of a limb: *Kalmia latifolia 200* in the same manner as above.

- Pain of great toe and joints with swelling, soreness, pain is more in warmth, by pressure, by motion and pain travels upwards: *Ledum palustre 200* in the same manner as above.

- Pains worse during rest, night and warmth, better by cold, open air and movement: *Pulsatilla nigricans 200* in the same manner as above.

▫ Pain, bruised and sprained, due to injury cannot bear touch: *Arnica montana 200* in the same above manner.

▫ Pain and nodosities (node is a protuberance or swelling) of joints: *Guajacum officinale 200* in the same above manner.

▫ Gouty pain complaints with offensive urine: *Acidum benzoicum 30* three times a day for seven days.

▫ Gouty pain complaints with red urine: *Lycopodium 200* one dose every third day, total three doses.

▫ Enlargement of joints, pain worse during rest and when storm approaches: *Rhododendron chrysanthum 200*, two times a day for three days.

▫ Gouty pain with high uric acid and urates: *Urtica uren-Q, 10* drops in half cup of water, three times a day for seven days.

▫ Arthritic deformans (when joints are deformed), particularly fingers: *Picricum acidum 200* weekly one dose for three weeks.

▫ Pains of joints or muscles with numbness: *Chamomilla 200* two times a day for three days in the same above manner.

▫ Pains appear diagonally, right arm and left leg, numbness and sensation of cold: *Agaricus muscarius 200* in the same above manner.

▫ Pains fly like electric shock, exposure to dampness, pains better by warmth: *Phytolacca decandra 200* in the same above manner.

▫ Rheumatic pains of joints worse after washing clothes: *Sepia officinalis 200* in the same above manner.

▫ Pain worse touch and when there has been loss of vital fluids: *China officinalis 30* three times a day for seven days.

- Pain heels better by putting most of weight over them: *Berberis vulgaris 200* two times a day for three days.

- Pain of heels and toes, swelling, coldness, stiffness, feverish feeling: *Colchicum autumnale 200* in the same above manner.

- Pain from elbow to hand, relieved by heat, pain at back: *Aesculus hippocastanum 200* in the same above manner.

- Pain arm to finger: *Chelidonium majus 200* as above.

- Pain arm to elbow or thumb to elbow: *Calcarea sulphurica 200* as above.

- Pain elbow, left: *Gelsemium sempervirens 200* as above.

- Pain elbow, right: *Oxalicum acidum 200* as above.

- Pain hip to knee (right), with swelling of knees: *Kalium carbonica 200* one dose only. Wait for three days.

- Pain in ribs, chest: *Bryonia alba 200*, two times a day for three days.

- Pains shifting: *Pulsatilla nigricans 200* as above.

- Pain sides lain on: *Phytolacca decandra 200* as above.

- Pain thighs: *Rhus toxicodendron 200* as above.

- Pain under thigh: *Phytolacca decandra 200*.

- Pain suddenly coming and suddenly disappearing: *Belladonna*, three times a day for three days.

- Pain gradually coming and gradually going: *Stannum metallicum*, as in the above manner.

- Pains, calves: *Lachesis mutus 200 as above.*

- Pain, ribs (right): *Borax veneta 200* as above.

- Pain in limbs and limbs give away while standing for a

long time or sitting for long time in ('Kirtan', 'Puja'): *Stannum metallicum 200*, one dose on alternate days, total three doses.

Aversions
KNOW ABOUT AVERSIONS ?

EVERYONE HAS his/her liking and disliking, desires and aversions. Someone likes to have apples every day; the others do not want to even smell it. A child licks the butter with his tongue. So compulsive is the desire. The other hates to see it, not even want to talk about eating it. This is aversion. Homoeopathy has a link with desires, aversions and modalities to verify the remedy to its totality with the totality of symptoms of disease. Until this is done, complete cure is doubtful in chronic diseases. To utilize this subject, here is an example. If some one is having abdominal pain and his symptoms are burning pains relieved by warm applications, digestive troubles after decayed food, non-vegetarian food, and alcohol, chewing tobacco, pains with restlessness and thirst for little water at a time and feeling of chilliness. The remedy is Ars. (See under 'Abdomen pain' heading) If the patient does not like to have cold water in addition to above abdominal symptoms, giving him Ars. is confirmed.

First Step Treatment: None

Special Note : All medicines are to be taken in 200 potency and in single dose. If found in favour, repeat the dose after fifteen days, otherwise consult a doctor.

Medicines

Aversion to:

▫   Potatoes: *Alumina.*

▫   Cheese: *Argentum nitricum.*

- Fish, salt, sugar: *Graphites.*
- Beer: *Nux vomica.*
- Ice cream: *Radium bromatum.*
- Milk, honey: *Natrium carbonicum.*
- Hot milk, onion, oranges, spices, pastry: *Phosphorus.*
- Apple: *Antimonium tartaricum.*
- Eggs: *Ferrum metallicum.*
- Pickles: *Abies nigra.*
- Coffee: *Psorinum.*
- Banana and plums: *Baryta carbonica.*
- Fruits: *Baryta carbonica.*
- Soup: *Rhus toxicodendron.*
- Cabbage, brandy: *Carbo vegetabilis.*
- Bread, butter, and hot food: *Natrium muriaticum.*
- Cold icy drinks: *Arsenicum album.*
- Cold water, garlic, onions, wine: *Sabadilla.*
- Vegetables: *Magnesium carbonicum.*

Awkward Behaviour (Mind)
KNOW ABOUT MIND AND AWKWARD BEHAVIOUR ?

WHAT IS life? Life can be identified in three dimensions. The mind, the body and the spirit or vital energy and without these three, unity of body cannot be defined. No two individuals are alike. Their body, mind and their energy differ. Each one has a special personality and special psychophysical structure and all this is decided by hereditary tendencies, social living habits and factor of diseases invading a person. Awkward behaviour can be easily identified in children and can also be seen in adults. This has a definite relation with diseases. Homoeopathy deals with individual while assessing their diseases, their habits, behaviours, likings, dislikings and so on. I cite an example. If the medicine you have selected for right- sided complaints and other symptoms of 'Lycopodium', check with him whether he shakes feet while sitting on chair. If so, Lycopodium is confirmed. On the other hand, if you find a person shaking his feet while sitting on chair, think of Lycopodium and then ask about his other ailments, for which he had come to you. The following data will act as clues to the medicines.

First Step Treatment: None

Special Note : All medicines are to be taken in 200 potency and in single dose. Repeat it after 15 days if results found in favour, otherwise consult a doctor.

Medicines

▫ Shakes feet while sitting on chair: *Lycopodium clavatum.*

▫ Confused, asks clarification about intake of medicine time again and again: *Lachesis mutus.*

▫ Cannot stand for long time, seeks chair: *Sulphur.*

▫ Keeps feet apart, while urinating: *Chimaphila umbellata.*

▫ Keeps hands moving on objects placed on the table, plays with his fingers: *Kalium muriaticum.*

▫ Sits reclining on chair, back and head must touch back of chair: *Magnesium phosphoricum.*

▫ Runs than walk: *Natrium muriaticum.*

▫ Uses two pillows under head: *Natrium muriaticum.*

▫ Always in a hurry: *Natrium phosphoricum.*

▫ Very religious: *Natrium sulphuricum.*

- Very shy: *Silicea terra.*

- Protudes tongue frequently: *Lachesis mutus.*

- Changes from one subject to other quickly: *Lachesis mutus.*

- Declares nothing the matter with him: *Arnica montana.*

- Avoids members of family: *Sepia officinalis.*

- Stumbling while walking: *Agaricus muscarius.*

- Drops things from hand: *Apis.*

- Angry when touched: *Tarentula hispanica.*

- Forgets or loses his way in well-known streets: *Glonoinum.*

- Winking eyes frequently: *Belladonna.*

- Sleeps with arms over head or abdomen: *Pulsatilla nigricans.*

- Pulls own hair: *Belladonna.*

- Irritated when questioned: *Nux vomica.*

- Sends doctor home saying he is not ill: *Arnica montana.*

Backache
KNOW ABOUT BACKACHE ?

BACKACHE IS called lumbago also. As the name indicates, it is pain in the back. No particular place in the back is assessed by the patient for pains and yet the pain exists somewhere. The pain comes in the way you use your body, carry weights, manage your diet and digestion power, your sexual frequency, and the method you adopt to erase your stress and worries. It is very common in both affluent and middle class and every one experiences it. In women it may be due to bad postures while cleaning floors and due to irregular menses. Reasons are many and so are the remedies.

First Step Treatment:

- If you sit on a computer, see that your knees are bent at an angle of ninety degree and that your lower back is supported by back of your chair.

- If you go for long drives on a car, see that your back is supported.

- If your stomach and abdomen muscles are strong, you will not have much of back problems. To make your abdominal muscles strong, you must do some mild abdominal exercises regularly.

- If you have a habit of taking prolonged rest, better join 'Yoga' classes to have a first step treatment.

- Massaging gently on both the sides of the spine with some mustard oil gives relief to pains.

- If the pain is sudden and severe and you feel numbness or loss of sensation in the back, contact the doctor immediately.

Medicines

- Sudden backache due to exposure to dry cold winds: *Aconitum napellus 30*, four times a day for three days.

- Due to exposure to cold, over exertion, worse initial movement and better continuous movement, worse rest: *Rhus toxicodendron 200*, two times a day for three days.

- With stiffness, worse movement and cold, better lying still: *Bryonia alba 200* in the above manner. Due to Injury: *Arnica montana 200* as above.

□ If the injury is on nerves: *Hypericum perforatum 30*, three times a day for three days.

□ Pricking pain, weakness and sweating, aggravation of pain at 3-4 a.m.: *Kalium carbonicum 200* only one dose. Wait for three days.

□ Backache of obese people, worse bathing and exposure to cold: *Calcarea carbonica 200* two times a day for three days.

□ Lower back pain, better sleep and rest, desire open air and cold: *Pulsatilla nigricans 200* as above.

□ Backache better by belching, chilly feeling: *Sepia officinalis 30*, four times a day for three days.

□ Chilly, constipated persons, pain worse cold, motion, turning in bed, has to sit up in bed and then turn in bed: *Nux vomica 200*, two times a day for three days.

□ Pain lower back due to constipation and piles, better only when standing: *Aesculus hippocastanum 200* in the above manner.

□ Backache worse damp cold places and bending for long hours: *Dulcamara 200* in the above manner.

□ Pain in lower back and coccyx, cannot walk erect, pain better in damp and cold but worse night, burning of soles: *Sulphur 200*, one dose in the morning for three days.

□ Pains back, neck, lumbao-sacral regions-down thighs, stiffness and contraction, spine sensitive with pain in scapula and right shoulder: *Cimicifuga racemosa 200*, two times a day for three days.

□ Pain worse while sitting, better by motion, itching and frozen feeling of toes and feet: *Chelidonium majus 200*, two times a day for three days.

□ More of pain in small of back and settles on upper part

of thigh and buttock. Patient limps and at last pain is so severe that he or she is unable to walk and stand, pains better pressure: *Colocynthis 200* two times a day for three days.

▫ Pain mostly comes in stormy weather: *Rhododendron chrysanthum 200* as above.

▫ Backache after excessive indulging in sex, worse in morning before rising: *Staphysagria 200* as above.

▫ Pain violent in upper back and then descend in lower back: *Kalmia latifolia 200* in the same above manner.

Bad or Offensive breath (Halitosis)
KNOW ABOUT OFFENSIVE BREATH ?

IF THERE is persistent bad breath, it is due to lack of oral hygiene. If your breath is bad, nobody would stand near you and would avoid too. Bad breath is the result of disorder of digestive system, pyorrhoea, bleeding gums, tooth decay, taking strongly flavoured foods like garlic, onions, smoking cigarette, chewing tobacco or taking cheap quality alcohol. Oral hygiene has to be maintained in the first instance. Please read my book, 'Oral Diseases' (page 189) published by M/s B. Jain Publishers, 1921, 10th street, Chuna Mandi, Paharganj, New Delhi 110055, for a detailed study.

First Step Treatment

● In case of tooth decay, mouth ulcers or gums bleeding, get proper treatment from doctor.

● Do not take non-vegetarian food and clean your mouth with tooth -pick after each such hard meal. Brush your teeth after each meal. Chew aniseed ('Saunf'), cardamom ('Chhoti Ilaichi') and clove ('Laung') after taking meals or keep either of them in mouth for sometime when you meet people.

- You should eat more of green and leafy vegetables. They contain chlorophyll, which prevents bad breath.

- If the bad breath continues for a longer time inspite of above steps, consult a doctor

Medicines

- Bad odour from mouth with excessive flow of saliva, corners of mouth cracked and raw feeling of palate: *Arum triphyllum 30*, three times a day for seven days.

- If the gums are swollen, bad breath, tongue and mouth are moist but still there is more of thirst: *Mercurius solubilis 30*, three times a day for seven days. Take the third dose before sun set.

- Bad odours due to pyorrhoea, gums are red and dark, bleeding and foetid salivation: *Baptisia tinctoria*, two times a day for seven days.

- Offensive breath, tooth decay and pain in teeth, gums ulcerated and bleeding: *Kreosotum*, three times a day for seven days.

- Gums sensitive to cold water, bad breath from mouth, boils on gums, caries of teeth and pyorrhoea: *Silicea terra*, two times a day for five days.

- Pyorrhoea, bad smell from mouth, gums swollen, purple and spongy, salivation, taste bitter and salty: *Mercurius corrosivus*, three times a day for seven days.

- Teeth black and crumbling, salivation, gums bleed easily, bad breath: *Staphysagria*, three times a day for seven days.

Bloating of Stomach

KNOW ABOUT BLOATING OF STOMACH ?

ONE OF the common ailments of the day is bloating or distention of the stomach or swelling of abdomen after eating. This may be due to excessive wind accumulation or fluid retention in the stomach or abdomen. The changed style of food habits is responsible for this problem. Old men and women are also prone to it because they eat more than their capacity. They do not reduce their intake with the increase of age. The young generation suffers from it due to intake of junk food, fast food and use of cold drinks in place of water. Business executive and service cadre people are always busy. They take food without proper chewing and are always in haste. Distension of abdomen is also felt in women who are about to menstruate. Hormonal changes sometimes retain the fluid and cause distention. Constipation, sensitivity to certain foods, especially milk, ulceration of intestinal lining and bacteria also causes bloating of abdomen.

First Step Treatment

- Chew your food completely before swallowing it. Never be in haste. Take enough of time during meals and be relaxed. Avoid viewing television during taking meals.

- Avoid taking excessive salt, non-vegetarian food, fried food, canned or frozen vegetables, sauce, pickles and soups.

- Have small and frequent food instead of taking a full meal.

- Avoid taking water with meals. Take water before or after half an hour of meals.

- Avoid taking too much cold drinks (carbonated beverages) and ice creams.

- Starchy foods like potatoes be avoided.

- Better keep one time fast in a week.

- If you are unable to digest milk (producing flatulence), do not take it.

●   Avoid taking too much of tea or coffee.

●   Avoid smoking or chewing tobacco.

●   When feeling too much bloating of abdomen, take tea containing ginger, cinnamon, aniseed and black pepper without milk.

Medicines

▫ Bloating of stomach as if there is a weight of stone: *Nux vomica 200* one dose weekly for three weeks.

▫ Wants to loosen the clothes after meals: *Pulsatilla nigricans 200* one dose weekly for two weeks.

▫ The wind in the stomach has a tendency to go upwards, discomfort in the chest: *Carbo vegetabilis 200* one dose weekly for three weeks.

▫ The wind in the stomach is passing downward: *Lycopodium clavatum* 30, three doses a day for two days. Take the last dose before seven in the evening. After ten days take *Lycopodium clavatum 200* one dose.

▫ The wind is accumulated in the stomach and is neither moving upwards nor downwards: *China officinalis 30,* three times a day for two days. After ten days, take *China officinalis 200* one dose.

Burns
KNOW ABOUT BURNS ?

BURNS ON the skin are due to exposure to heat, electricity and chemicals. Most of the burns take place in kitchen and on the day of 'Diwali', when crackers do the mischief. If a prompt home treatment is taken, the intensity of burns can be reduced and doctor at hospital will find it easy to promote healing. If the burns are not deep, they will be cured by homoeopathy and taking following measures.

F- 8

First Step Treatment

• An immediate attention is needed to take care of burns. If the burns are due to short circuit of electricity or due to chemicals, it will be deep burns and first duty is to take the patient to the doctor.

• When the dress of a person catches fire, push him or her to the floor since flames always mount upwards. Now take a blanket, tablecloth, rug, bedsheet or a coat, whatever is available nearby, and throw over the flames pressing the cloth well down in all the directions. Many frightful burns can thus be avoided in this way.

• As soon as the burns due to fire takes place, put the area of burn under running cold water for at least 5 to 10 minutes.

• If some jewellery or rings cover the area of burn, remove them. If clothing is there, remove it too.

• If blisters have come up at the area of burns, do not break them.

• If the area of burn is more than seven centimeters, the burn is deeper than the upper skin, if the burns are on face, mouth, near eyes or throat, take the patient to the doctor immediately.

Medicines

▫ If there are no blisters, the burns are confined to the skin, apply Urtica ointment. Internally, take *Cantharis*, three times a day for five days.

▫ If the blisters have come up, take *Cantharis vesicatoria* orally, three times a day for five days.

▫ If after burns, the wounds have come up, apply *Calendula* ointment. Take *Cantharis vesicatoria* orally three times a day for five days.

▫ If the patient is very much under shock or fear due to burns, give two doses of Aconitum napellus at the interval of 15 minutes and then give *Cantharis vesicatoria* for two times on the day of burn. *Cantharis vesicatoria* is to be continued three times a day for six days.

▫ If the burns are very deep and skin is destroyed, give *Kalium bichromicum*, four times a day for one day and take the patient to doctor.

New opinion about handling burns

Some people had an idea that holding ice against the burns and applying ghee or butter gives speedy recovery. Some experts have viewed this method differently now. They say that ghee or butter will retain the heat of burns inside the skin and applying ice may damage tissues further. The best is to remove any sticking of clothing etc. on the burns and then flush the area of burn in cold running water for some minutes. Soaking in water for another 20 to 30 minutes will help relieve the pains.

Boils
KNOW ABOUT BOILS ?

BOILS ON the skin are eruptions, which are painful, deep red colour, tender and painful terminated in suppuration. Boils are lumps containing pus as well. The cause is bacterial and disordered condition of the blood, as a result of improper, indigestible food and anxiety. If boils recur frequently, this may be due to weakness of the immune system. They come up in the skin around a hair follicle. The most common sites of boils are face, neck, armpits and groin. Boil is visible on the skin and if it is beneath the skin but show tender swelling, it is called abscess. Boils and abcesses generally come to head, contain a sac of pus, discharge pus and subside.

First Step Treatment

- Eruption of boils, once a year or upon change of season is a process of making the system immune. Do not panic and take it lightly.

- When you see that suppuration is taking place, keep a poultice covered with oiled layer of cloth. (Preferrably mustard oil) The poultice should be kept hot and renewed until suppuration is nearly completed. The poultice can also be that of hot onion, mustard oil and 'Haldi'.

- Do not press the boil to burst it *yourself.* It may spread the infection.

- Take a piece of garlic every day in the morning.

Medicines

- The first remedy of boils when they appear and are red, painful: *Belladonna*, three times a day for four days.

- In the beginning of suppuration when pus is developing: *Hepar sulphur*, three doses a day for one day. This will hasten suppuration. If *Hepar sulphur* 200, one dose is given, it will check suppuration.

- When the boil does not heal although suppuration has taken place and the maturity of boil has not come up, give *Silicea terra*, three times day for two days.

- Very red boils, hot skin, shining and burning and there is fever also: *Aconitum napellus*, three times a day for three days.

- Very small boils in plenty scattered over body (summer boils): *Arnica montana 200.*

- When the boil is of long standing big, open and is full of pus, to absorb this pus, give *Mercurius solubilis* 200, one dose every third day in the morning, total three days. Also give *Gunpowder 3x*, four times a day for twelve days.

Cervical Spondylosis

KNOW ABOUT CERVICAL SPONDYLOSIS ?

CERVICAL SPONDYLOSIS is a condition pertaining to degeneration of the intervertebral discs. Neck pain is the product of cervical spondylosis and is due to very fast life, mechanical routine, lack of exercise, bad postures while sitting or sleeping and tensions besides the injuries. Neck pain is not due to one specific reason. (Please read my book, 'Manage and Cure Neck Pain, Cervical Spondylosis' for detailed study. Publishers: Health Harmony, 1921, Chuna Mandi, Paharganj, New Delhi 110 055).

Note : Please see 'Neck-pain' on page 114 of this book.

Children Disorders

BED-WETTING

Know about Bed-Wetting ?

BED-WETTING or enuresis is the disorder of the children in which they urinate while in sleep. This may be due to irritation by the worms, intake of too large quantity of fluids, improper food and drink, resulting in acrid urine and constitutional weakness. As a matter of fact, the cause is obscure and mostly needs professional treatment. It has also physical as well as psychological reasons behind the complaint. In some cases, it is weakness of the bladder and in most of the cases it is due to some sort of fear or stress. For a child wetting the bed upto the age of three and half years, no medicine should be given. The size of their bladder and its capacity, the slow reflex command of the brain to express urge for urination to the organ and deep sleep are the natural traits of the body up to the stated age. Children who continue this habit even at the age of four and above, need a check up and medicines.

First Step Treatment

- Treat the child psychologically first. Never tell about his or her wetting the bed in presence of friends and relatives.

- Do not scold or rebuke the children for the bed wetting since it is not intentional. It is not their fault.

- A study is needed to find out whether the parents are fighting with each other in presence of the children.

- No punishment should be given to the child for wetting the bed.

- Hang a calender in the child's room and encircle the date in the calender with a red pen when the child wets the bed. This should be done in presence of child. This will enable you know the days, he or she wets the bed and make aware the child as well.

- Do not give milk to drink at bed- time to the child. Give it in the evening preferably with a 'chhuara' (dried date) boiled with milk.

- Reduce the intake of fluids, especially warm drinks, after 8 P.M., at least two hours before bedtime.

Medicines

- If child has habit of boring nose frequently, with itching at anus, white patches on face, grinds teeth in sleep, think that he or she has worms and bed wetting can also be due to worms: *Cina* 30, three times a day for six days.

- Bed wetting during first hour of sleep: *Causticum* 200 weekly one dose for three weeks.

- Wets the bed immediately after going to bed: *Sepia officinalis* 200 in the same above manner.

- Physical and psychological cause: *Equisetum hyemale* 30, three times a day for seven days.

- Bed-wetting and child complains of urine-burning: *Verbascum thapsus* 30, in the same above manner.

- Child gets the dreams of urination and does it: *Kreosotum* 30 in the same above manner.

- Child eats earth, lime, chalk etc (PICA) and also has bed-wetting: *Calcarea carbonica* 200, weekly for three weeks.

Note : It is better that the treatment should be under a homoeopath after one week, telling him the medicine, you have given.

STAMMERING

Consult a doctor for treatment after giving one dose of one of the following medicine as per symptoms.

Try this at home for stammering

APPLY ON the tongue of child a pinch of mountain salt ('sendha namak') mixed with cow-ghee daily for 15 days and see the result. Many a times this works if the tongue is thick.

First Step Treatment : None

Medicines

- Child exerts to speak: *Stramonium 200* one dose weekly, three weeks

- When Stram. fails, try: *Hyoscyamus niger 200* same as above.

- Specific for stammering: *Bovista lycoperdon 200*, same as above

- Stammering due to excitement: *Causticum 200*, same as above

- Child stammers due to thick tongue: *Natrium carb. 30*, three times daily for ten days.

- Stammers at words like X, S, V, T, A and P: *Lachesis mutus 200*, one dose weekly for three weeks.

ANOREXIA [NO APPETITE]

First Step Treatment : None

Medicines

- Hungry without appetite: *China officinalis 200*, weekly one dose , total two weeks.

- Hungry without appetite and vomiting after eating: *Ferrum metallicum 30*, three times a day for one week.

- No hunger but likes and takes excessive salt: *Natrium muriaticum 200*, one dose every week for two weeks.

- Hunger lost, child complains of pain in right side of stomach: *Chelidonium majus 200*, same as above.

VOMITING

Note : Giving a dose of one of the following medicines as per symptoms after each vomiting give better results.

First Step Treatment : None

Medicines

- Vomiting but the tongue is clean: Ipecac.30, 3 times a day for two days.

- Vomiting but the tongue white coated: *Antimonium crudum* 30, same as above.

- Vomiting after eating: *Aethusa cynapium* 30, same as above.

- Vomiting after eating but with great debility: *Ferrum metallicum* 30, same as above.

- Motor sickness, vomiting during journeys: *Cocculus indica* 30, three times a day for one day when on journey.

- Vomiting with pain in stomach: *Nux vomica* 30, three times a day for two days.

CONSTIPATION

First Step Treatment : None

Medicines

- First stool hard and then loose: *Calcarea carbonica* 200 in the morning.

- Small quantity of stool: *Nux vomica* 200 at bedtime.

- Hard and knotty stool, anus red, pain in abdomen, frequent desire: *Sulphur* 200 in the morning.

- Dry stool, great thirst: *Bryonia alba* 200 in the night.

- Dry crumbling stool: *Natrium muriaticum* 200 in the night

- Missing for days: *Alumina* 200 in the morning

Note : Give only one dose and watch the results for four days. In case of slight improvement, give another dose after a week of first dose. If no improvement after two doses, consult the doctor.

FEVER SIMPLE
Method of Management

Give medicine four times a day. In high fever more than 102 degree F, place cloth wet with cold water on the head and forehead. Along with this, immerse your hands in cold water and wet the backside of neck and wrists of the child with gentle touch. Do this for four to five times. Similarly after four or five wet cloth compress, note the temperature of the child and even if it has come down by half a degree, discontinue further cold compress and wetting the neck etc. The temperature will now come down by itself. Do not give a water bath to the child as it may abruptly drop the temperature, which is not required. If temperature is not coming down even after cold-water compress, 'crocin' or 'nimulid' (in tablet or liquid form) can be given. Lowering of temperature is the prime motive. Forget about use of homoeopathic or allopathic medicines at this juncture. Give the child lot of water to drink so that he urinates or sweats frequently. Give him or her light meals like milk with bread, 'khichri' (rice and gram), 'Dalia' or 'roti' without 'ghee' with 'moong dhuli daal'.

Medicines

- First stage, exposure to hot or cold, chill, thirst is more: *Aconitum napellus* 30, four times a day for three days. Reduce the dose to three times a day for next two days and then to two doses a day for two days and last one dose a day for one day.

- Fever due to change of weather: *Arsenicum album* 30, same as above.

- High fever without thirst, head hot, feet cold: *Belladonna* 30, same as above.

- With muscular pains, chill down the spine, no thirst: *Gelsemium sempervirens* 30, same as above.

▫ With gastric derangement, chilly but wants no covering: *Nux vomica* 30, same as above.

▫ With restlessness and bodyache: *Rhus toxicodendron* 30, same as above.

CHILDREN-NORMAL WEIGHT OTHER NORMS [AVERAGE]

● At birth: 3.2 kg

● 4th month: 6.5 kg.

● One year: 9.7 kg.

● 6th year: 18.6 kg.

● Head measurement:
Birth: 32.5 cm.,
9th month: 42.5 cm,
one year: 45 cm

● Teething:
6 months, complete by 3 years,
New teething: 6th to 12th year.

● (The measures vary according to lean, medium or strong built of the child and only doctor can tell whether your child is under or over weight)

Colic of Babies
KNOW ABOUT COLIC ?

COLIC STANDS for pain in the stomach or abdomen region. To the babies, colic means bouts of crying that are inconsolable. The infants (mostly upto the age of four months) get rid of this colic by getting tuned to the feed and environment. The baby cries for long time, even upto an hour or so, now and then, mostly in the evening or night. The knees are drawn up to chest and if you feel the stomach, it will be felt hard or distended. The crying of baby has to be distinguished from that of cries for hunger. In hunger, the spell of crying is not long. The underlying reasons behind colic are not fully known but there are many possible explanations. Most of the infants having colic are otherwise found healthy.

First Step Treatment

- When the infants are breast-fed, it is first duty of the mothers to be careful about their diet. Change your diet to simple one. Mothers should not take hard indigestible food, non-vegetarian food, eggs, banana, chocolate, coffee, tinned stuff, fast food and packed dairy items.

- When the baby is crying, hold him or her against your chest so that his head is on your shoulder. Walk around giving pats on his back and singing some baby-song. Feeling secured, he will stop crying for some time.

- There is controversy over giving 'gripe water' and 'Janam ghutti' to the infants and many doctors of the conventional system do not recommend them. Think of these Indian traditional tonics for upkeep of babies and avoiding their gastric and colic problems. These are time- tested. Mothers throughout the countryside and cities have been giving 'gripe water' since times immemorial. I have not seen any adverse effect of giving these tonics.

- If the baby is not on mother's feed, give him aniseed water in milk. Put one teaspoonful of aniseed (saunf) in a cup of water in the night. In the morning, filter the water through a clean cloth and crush the aniseed by squeezing the cloth. A spoon full of this water mixed in a bottle of milk will remove flatulence and avoid colic.

- Application of water mixed with asafoetida (heeng) around the naval area gives instant relief to colic of babies. This is also a time- tested remedy.

- To avoid colic of the babies, it is better to give a massage to the baby everyday. With some mustard oil on the palms, gently massage the abdomen with slow movement of hand in clockwise fashion.

Medicines

- Mix 10 tablets of *Magnesia phosphorica* 6x in one-fourth cup of lukewarm water. Give half to one spoon of this water every five minutes; three to four doses will remove the colic of infants' upto the age of four months.

- In case of no relief, mix *Chamomilla*, two drops in half cup of water and dosage.

- Still no relief, mix *Colocynthis* two drops in the same above manner and dosage.

Common Colds (Coryza)
KNOW ABOUT COLDS ?

THE PICTURE of common cold is very much familiar to all. It starts with nose running, sneezing, watering of eyes, constriction in throat, desire to spit or swallow, hoarse voice, headache, pain in body, loss of appetite and slight rise in temperature of body. All the symptoms may not be present in the beginning and the most teasing part of the disorder is teasing discomfort. This annoying cold has many viruses in the background, which are fought with by our immune system. Mostly people get cold in winter. Children get cold more because of insufficient building of resistance in their bodies.

There is no fixed treatment known to cure cold immediately. It takes its own time of two to seven days according to the resistance of the individual to the infections.

First Step Treatment

- In two cups of water, mix some jaggery ('Gurh') and dried ginger ('Saunth') in it and boil the water till it is reduced to one cup. Filter the water with cloth and drink it when it is lukewarm, slowly sip by sip and not in a hurry.

- In a cup of lukewarm water, squeez one lemon-juice and half teaspoonful of honey and drink it thrice a day.

- Drinking some lukewarm water mixed with some salt, four to five times a day, sip by sip like tea, also brings relief to cold.

- Applying a coating of mustard oil inside the nostrils during daytime decreases the intensity of cold.

- Take plenty of rest on bed. Moving around in public places and on your business during colds reduces the body's resistance and makes one more susceptible to infections.

- Applying 'vicks' over the chest, back and around neck at bedtime gives some relief.

- Wash your hands frequently with antibacterial soap so that further germs do not contact with nose and mouth.

- Some experts also advise eating spicy food during cold. This helps nose to start more of discharge and acts as natural decongestant.

- Take plenty of liquids, water, soup, juice when cold cough is accompanied by fever.

Medicines

□ If the cold is due to exposure to cold winds, there is headache, sneezing and watering of eyes, feverish feeling and anxiety of getting more of illness, take *Aconitum napellus* 30, six times a day for one day. Reduce the dose to four times a day, the next day. Further reduce the dose three times day, the third day and then stop.

□ If there is bland discharge from the eyes and acrid discharge from nose, cold is better in open but worse in warmth, take *Allium cepa* 30 in the same above manner.

□ If the discharge from eyes is acrid and from nose it is bland, opposite to *Allium cepa*, take *Euphrasia officinalis* 30 in the same above manner.

□ If the discharge is acrid both from nose and eyes with restlessness and unquenchable thirst for little water at a time, take *Arsenicum album* 30 four times a day on the first day and three times a day for next two days.

□ If there is sense of weight in the forehead, nose closure at night but discharge of nose during day, take *Nux vomica 30* in the same above manner.

□ Severe cold with more of sneezing, redness of nose, pain in forehead and watering of eyes, take *Sabadilla 30* in the same above manner.

□ If the discharge from nose is thick and bland, there is pain and chilliness in the back, sneezing and patient is dull and lazy: give *Gelsemium sempervirens* 30, four times a day for three days.

□ When the first phase of cold is over and the discharge from nose and throat is thick and yellow with loss of smell and taste is bitter or no taste: Take *Pulsatilla nigricans* 30, three times a day for seven days.

Constipation

KNOW ABOUT CONSTIPATION ?

CONSTIPATION IS the disorder of inactive persons who do not bother to exercise and have sedentary jobs.

When you do not pass stool or there is infrequent bowel movement, you feel that there is something left in the abdomen or it is not clear, such condition is called constipation. This disorder is increasing day by day in India due to people indulging in fast food and preference to weekend dinners at hotels. With constipation, you will be restless, feel uneasiness and may pass gas frequently. If constipation is ignored, the condition leads to haemorrhoids (piles), which means that there is underlying intestinal disease. Constipation can also lead you to headaches, fatigue and bad breath.

First Step Treatment:

- Change your life-style in eating and water drinking.

- Take lot of green vegetables and fruits having high fibre.

- Avoid going to restaurants, taking fast food or junk food, taking fried and heavy meals.

- Take a glass of apple juice each day, if possible.

- Start morning or evening walks with some light exercises.

- Take at least two glasses of water after you get up from bed in the morning. Take one glass of milk every night before going to sleep.

- Increase your intake of water per day.

Medicines

☐ Sedentary life, ineffectual urging, passing stool many

times a day: *Nux vomica* 200, two times a day for three days.

□   Hard stool, dryness, desire for dry food: *Alumina* 200 (Better for old persons and children), in the same above manner.

□   Stool hard, dry, burnt, too large, no desire, thirst more at long intervals: *Bryonia alba* 200 in the same above manner.

□   Patient feels better and normal when constipated, fat, flabby, chilly patients: *Calcarea carbonica* 30, three times a day for seven days.

□   Constipated but can pass stool only when in standing position: *Causticum* 200 weekly one dose for three weeks.

□   Chronic constipation of old people with sinking feeling in stomach, tongue flabby and white: *Hydrastis canadensis* Q. Take 8 drops in half cup of water, twice daily for 7 days.

□   In chilly patients, stool goes back into rectum, when partially expelled: *Silicea terra* 200, weekly one dose for three weeks.

Cough
KNOW ABOUT COUGH ?

COUGH IS a common disorder and there is nothing to worry about if the cough does not persist for longer periods. This does not mean that medicine is not to be taken. A common cold, flu or an allergic reaction can cause infection of upper respiratory infection. Cough may be dry or with mucus. Actually, cough is a reflex action to clear the irritants and phlegm from the air passage. It is a process to clear respiratory tract. It also shows that the body has resistance to expel irritants from the breathing (respiratory) system. The pollution in the atmosphere, the exhausts of vehicles, the mucus or coryza going down from nasal cavity to throat and then irritating the air passage, any type of allergy any viral or bacterial infection in the passage due to above reasons, are some of the causes for simple cough. Cough is most common in winter and in areas where some kind of pollution exists.

First Step Treatment

- Avoid going to polluted areas and if you are a smoker, leave smoking.

- Take plenty of water during the day and prefer to drink luke-warm water at least three times a day.

- Avoid taking banana and curd.

- In winter cough, take a spoon full of honey with four drops of ginger ('adarak' in Hindi) or Onion juice every day twice or thrice daily.

- If the cough is of barking, rough and harsh nature, (called croup here), inhaling steam is useful. Keep a kettle of boiling water near you on the floor and sit covering your head and kettle with a big towel. Besides this method, electric vaporizers are also available in the market.

- Gently massage the chest, back and neck of the patient with lukewarm garlic-mustard oil. To prepare this oil, put 4 small pieces (branches) from one full size garlic in one table spoonfull of mustard oil and heat it up to the point when garlic is about to burn or becomes brownish red. Allow it to cool down to lukewarm temperature and then apply this oil by removing garlic pieces. After gentle massaging of chest, back and neck areas of the patient, do not allow the patient to get exposed to cold air. Better do this just before the patient goes to bed for sleeping.

Medicines

□ Cough on account of exposure of cold winds and when the patient is too much worried or afraid of the cough: *Aconitum napellus 30* four times a day for one day and then three times a day for next two days.

□ Cough brings pain in distant part of body, throat burning: *Capsicum annuum 30*, three times a day for three days.

□ Feels sleepy after coughing in spasms, cough increases desire for more coughing, much of sighing, patient mentally or physically exhausted: *Ignatia amara 30* in the same above manner.

□ Cough at night with oppression of chest, cough coming deep from the chest and cough at night with diarrhoea during day: *Petroleum 30* in the same above manner.

□ Cough during inspiration and during night, breathing in cool air at night and dry cough, tickling in throat bring cough: *Rumex crispus 30* in the same above manner.

□ Spell of cough ends in sneezing, difficulty in raising tough profuse mucus in the aged, pain in the back on coughing: *Senega-Q*, ten drops in half cup of water three times a day for three days.

□ Cough causes pain in chest and headache, stools dry with constipation, thirst more: *Bryonia alba 30* four times a day for three days.

□ Cough with hoarseness, loss of voice, likes icy cold water even in cough: *Phosphorus 200* one dose in the morning and one dose in the morning on third day.

□ Cough with feeling as if there is dust in throat, small lumps of mucus fly out of mouth when coughing, alternate diarrhoea and constipation with cough: *Chelidonium majus 30*, three times a day for three days.

- Pain in ears when coughing, phlegm is sticky, ropy: *Kalium bichromicum 30* in the same above manner.

- Cough comes at 3 a.m: *Kalium carbonicum 200* one dose in the morning and one dose on fourth day, if there is no improvement. No repetition if the relief comes after one dose. Wait for the results for four days after one day of taking first dose.

- Cough comes in warm room, better in open air, thirst less with dry mouth: *Pulsatilla nigricans 30*, three times a day for three days.

- Dry cough with hissing sounds as if saw is driven, wheezing, sensation of plug in the throat, great dryness of air pasages: *Spongia tosta 30*, four times a day for one day and three times a day for next three days.

- With coughing, urine escapes, dry cough better in cold damp weather, scanty expectoration, must be swallowed: *Causticum 200*, one dose daily for three days.

- Cough worse after first sleep and with wheezing, tongue clean, at times nausea and vomiting: *Ipecac uanha 30*, three times a day for three days.

- Rattling of chest with phlegm that is difficult to expel, tongue white coated, coughing and yawning alternate: *Antimonium tartaricum 30* three times a day for three days.

- Cough dry at night, tickling, short, choking, face red on coughing, larynx very painful, high piping voice: *Belladonna 30*, four times a day for three days.

- Exposure to cold wind with sensation of foreign body in throat, pain during swallowing, sensitive to touch, cough is more when exposed to cold, choking cough: *Hepar sulphur 30*, three times a day for three days. The phlegm will be now released easily. On fourth day, no medicine and then take one dose of *Hepar sulphur* 200 on fifth day.

□ Cough with itching in larynx, spasmodic cough with burning in the chest, hoarseness, wheezing, vomiting, cough after diseases, cough with flatulence: *Carbo vegetabilis 30* three times a day for three days.

□ Phlegm yellow and sweet, weakness and emptiness in chest: *Stannum metallicum 30* in the same above manner.

□ Dry cough, has to stoop to cough, constipation with cough: *Kalium muriaticum 30* in the same above manner.

□ Child crying before and during coughing, violent cough with facial herpes, cough worse exercise and during night: *Arnica montana 200*, one dose a day for three days.

Note : If the cough does not improve after five days, consult a homoeopath

Cramps In Legs
KNOW ABOUT CRAMPS IN LEGS ?

CRAMPS IN Hindi is 'Bayte'that is a extremely painful condition of muscles of legs.

The patients cry and get on the verge of weeping due to severe and sudden muscle Spasm that gives severe pains. The cramp is mostly in the leg (calf) muscles but it can be on arm, hand or foot too. It occurs occasionally but if it occurs every other day, the treatment is needed. It is mostly experienced during sleeping sessions. During sleeping, when legs are stretched in a straightened position or given an awkward jerk without one knows, the cramps occur. Cramps are due to contraction of muscles and cause damage of nerves due to poor circulation of blood or adopting some wrong awkward postures of sitting and standing.

First Step Treatment

- After getting a cramp, try to move toes of the affected leg to and fro in lying position, keeping leg touched with bed.

- Now sit on the bed and press the middle of the back of calf (meeting point of muscles and tendon) with your thumb.

- Keep the pressure of thumb constantly and start moving the thumb upwards towards the joint of knee.

- When the pain is little less, cup your legs with both hands and press inwards side of legs from calf to knee.

- Application of hot compress also helps removing the cramp.

- When slight pain remains for a long time, apply *Arnica* ointment.

- The best prevention for recurrence of cramps is to take lot of water and less of salt.

Medicines

- Cramps in the muscles of calf at night while stretching: *Rhus toxicodendron 30*, three doses at the interval of 5 minutes during attack. Take the same medicine three times a day on the next day.

- Cramps recurring in calf muscles or in muscles of soles, palms, toes and fingers, take *Cuprum metallicum 30*, three times a day for five days.

- Cramps due to excessive tiredness and fatigue and one feels as if bruised: *Arnica montana 30*, three times a day for three days.

Cravings (Desires)
KNOW ABOUT CRAVINGS ?

CRAVING IS desire for eatable and other things. You must have seen simple cases of children eating chalk, chewing pencils, eating papers, slates etc. Similarly, there are people who would add more of salt or sugar in their eatables. Some people cannot take food without the help of pickles. Some take raw rice. Someone would like to have eggs every day without fail. All these are rated as cravings. Excess of everything is bad. There ought to be some adverse effects on the body. Even if such effects are not seen immediately, homoeopathy considers such desires or even aversions important and it helps find out a medicine. If somebody is having a problem with digestion and he has a craving for salt, it hints towards the medicine nat-m. Let the body give any symptoms, *nat-m.* should be tried. Of course, a good doctor would always go by the other symptoms of nat-m. A layman can also give a dose of nat-m. to a person having craving for salt and might see miraculous results.

First Step Treatment: None
Medicines for some of the cravings:

Desire or craving for:

- Cloth, raw food, raw rice: *Alumina 200.*

- Fat, lime, slate, pencils, chalk, clay etc.: *Acidum nitricum 200.*

- Salt: *Natrium muriaticum 200.*

- Eggs: *Calcarea carbonica 200.*

- Sweets: *Argentum nitricum 200.*

- Pickles and sour foods: *Sepia officinalis 200.*

- Lemonade: *Pulsatilla nigricans 200.*

- Banana: *Theridion 200.*

- Icy cold drinks, fond of, always wants: *Phosphorus 200.*

- Milk: *Rhus toxicodendron 200.*

- Wants everything cold: *Secale cornutum 200.*

Note : Only one dose is to be taken. Wait for the results for 15 days and if found in favour, repeat one dose. If there is no relief, consult a doctor.

Dandruff

KNOW ABOUT DANDRUFF ?

Dandruff is a common skin disease of the scalp and hair. There are thin dry scales (dead skin), which peel off from the scalp without any prior inflammation. It creates itching and irritation. The young generation of cities and big towns has this problem due to no application of oil and frequent use of shampoos containing chemicals. Lured by TV commercials and advertisements, they leave their hair dry without oil and invite dandruff. Just think, if pollution and dirt can harm lungs, why not skin? The dirt that falls on the dry hair is not obstructed by hair and it reaches the roots causing irritation and debris of dust go on accumulating. If the hair have some oil, the dirt would be sticking to the hair and may not reach the scalp. It is the city where more of people are having this problem. In rural areas, dandruff is not even known.

First Step Treatment

- Wash the hair at least thrice in a week (females) and daily for males. Do not use hard shampoo containing chemicals. Use herbal shampoo or soap containing shikakai, 'amla' or glycerine.

- Use your own clean comb and brush and do not use

combs or brushes of others.

- In summer, use curd for washing the hair. Apply curd on the hair and wash the hair after 15-20 minutes.

- Apply fresh lemon juice on the scalp and wash after 20 minutes.

Medicines

☐ Whole scalp is covered with dandruff and hair fall in bunches: *Phosphorus 200*, one dose a week. Take a total of two doses.

☐ Dandruff with itching, which is worse when bathing with hot water, at times there is headache also: *Lycopodium clavatum 200* in the same above manner.

☐ Dandruff with itching but it is in dry scales coming out when scratched, scalp is sensitive and patient takes little water at a time instead of taking full glass of water: *Arsenicum album 200* in the same above manner.

☐ Dandruff white, scaly, hair dry, falling of hair, is more in damp weather: *Thuja occidentalis 200* in the same above manner.

☐ Dandruff more on margin of hair, skin is oily, patient craves for salt: *Natrium muriaticum 200* in the same above manner.

☐ Abundant dandruff, scaly, with frequent sweat on back of head (occiput): *Sanicula aqua 200*, in the same above manner.

☐ Dandruff in circular patches like ringworms, itching not relieved by scratching, patient feels lot of weakness and if female, her periods are irregular: *Sepia officinalis 200* in the same above manner.

☐ Dandruff with pain felt in the roots of hair, head and forehead has more of sweating: *Calcarea carbonica 200* in the same above manner.

Diarrhoea
KNOW ABOUT DIARRHOEA?

COMMON DIARRHOEA is a functional disorder having frequent watery evacuation without inflammation of the intestines. Diarrhoea is about having loose motions a number of times when there is improper digestion and food gradients travel faster than the required rate for digestion in the digestive canal. The reason is some infection. Even if no medicine is given to the patient and complete rest is taken with more intake of fluids, the diarrhoea gets cured. If diarrhoea lasts for a few days, it may be as a result of food poisoning created by some bacterial or viral infections along the lining of stomach and intestines. Many a times, diarrhoea is due to intolerance to certain foods like milk, cream, cheese, meat etc. It may also be due to side effect of too many medicines, taking excessive, indigestible unripe, decayed fruits, diseased animal food, atmospheric influences, fatigue, suppressed skin disease and mental emotions. One must remember that diarrhoea due to indigestion is an effort of the body-system to expel substances that might otherwise give serious troubles.

First Step Treatment

- Take plenty of rest on the bed. Better lie down for some hours.

- Avoid sudden changes of temperature.

- Physical excesses and mental strain should be avoided.

- Plenty of boiled water mixed with sugar and a pinch of salt should be taken.

- Taking Electral or ORS solution, (WHO recommended) also helps.

- Tea, coffee, eggs, meat, spices, fruits and stimulants should be avoided.

- Take two teaspoonful of 'Isabgol' (Plantago ovata) mixed with curd and sugar, two times a day.

- In meals take rice and curd.

- After meals, take one teaspoonful of 'Saunf'(Aniseed) with 'Mishri'.

- Avoid travelling and taking meals in the hotels during attack of diarrhoea.

- Wash hands with soap thoroughly after every evacuation and wipe them clean. Keep a separate towel for the patient. Avoid going to public toilets for evacuation.

Note : If the diarrhoea is not cared for and one develops symptoms of dehydration i.e. drowsiness, scanty urine, restlessness and vomiting, consult the doctor immediately.

Medicines

□ Summer diarrhoea due to over eating of fruits, painless motions after eating, morning or night with weakness, thirst, loss of appetite, stool gush out with force: *China officinalis 30*, six doses a day preferably after every evacuation till there is improvement. If there is improvement after three or four doses, stop taking the medicine. Take the medicine two times next day and the third day for once only.

□ Loose motions due to exposure of cold, and dampness, chilly feelings, thirst more and feeling feverish: *Aconitum napellus 30* in the same above manner.

□ Diarrhoea of children, hot, greenish, painful, during dentition, child screams and is irritable: *Chamomilla* in the same manner.

□ Due to late night eating, drinking and over eating: *Nux vomica 30* in the same manner as above.

- After every stool, there is burning, restlessness, weakness, stool of foul smell, much thirst, loose motions due to eating stale food, fish, meat or milk or stale vegetables, ice-cream or acids: *Arsenicum album 30* in the same above manner.

- Diarrhoea profuse, gushing out with force, better after sleeping and stool with white particles like boiled sago: *Podophyllum peltatum 30* in the same above manner.

- Yellow, foetid stools, evacuation follows quickly upon urging for them, pain in the pelvis before and during evacuation, morning diarrhoea urging wakens the patient driving the patient out of bed and stool with passage of flatus: *Aloes socotrina 30* in the same above manner.

If you know the cause of diarrhoea following medicines will work better

Drinking contaminated water: *Chamomilla 30.*

Exposure to cold in rainy season: *Dulcamara 30.*

Drinking milk: *Aethusa cynapium 30.*

Eating fatty food: *Pulsatilla nigricans 30.*

Exposure to heat in day and cold at night: *Bryonia alba 30.*

Due to getting news of joy: *Coffea cruda 30.*

Due to getting news of grief: *Ignatia amara 30.*

Diarrhoea after delivery of baby: *China officinalis 30.*

After taking too much fruits: *China officinalis 30.*

Taking ice-cream or ice: *Arsenicum album 30.*

Note : These medicines are to be taken in the above manner as shown against symptom-wise medicines.

Directional and Diagonal Symptoms
KNOW ABOUT DIAGONAL SYMPTOMS?

JUST LIKE aversions and desires, diagonal and directional symptoms of disease help in selecting proper medicines. These are peculiar symptoms and many a times, these are very helpful. You need not go in for other symptoms of the disease and only one dose of the medicine in 200 potency is to be taken. Repeat it after 7 days; if there is relief. Wait for another 3 days and then consult a doctor.

First Step Treatment : None

Medicines

Diagonal and directional pains

- Pain in upper left arm and lower right leg: Agaricus muscarius.

- Upper right organ and lower left organ: Ambra grisea

- Pain travelling downwards, say shoulder to hand or thigh to leg: Kalmia latifolia.

- Pain travelling upwards, say hand to shoulder or foot to leg to thigh: Ledum palustre.

- Pain shifting from left side to right side: Lachesis mutus.

- Pain shifting from right side to left side: Belladonna

- Symptoms changing sides frequently: Lacaninum.

Debility or Weakness
KNOW ABOUT DEBILITY?

DEBILITY IS weakness and this may be due to many causes. Deficiency in diet, low blood pressure, anaemic conditions, effects of taking too many medicines, after diarrhoea, after profuse menses, after excessive exercises or too much of household work without taking rest, mental worries and tension are some of the important causes of weakness. In northern India, the elders advice for good vegetarian diet and milk to erase weakness. Given here are some medicines which may overcome weakness but if the same persists, doctor should be consulted. Take the medicine in 30th potency three times a day for seven days.

First Step Treatment : None

Medicines

Weakness from ascending stairs: *Calcarea phosphorica.*

From diarrhoea: *China officinalis.*

From slight movement: *Bryonia alba.*

Before menses: *Calcarea carbonica.*

After menses: *China officinalis.*

From sweating: *Bryonia alba.*

From talking or laughing: *Stannum metallicum.*

Earache or Ear Pain
KNOW ABOUT EARACHE?

EARACHE IS pain in ears. Most of the pains come after direct exposure to cold air, imperfect drying of the ear after taking a bath or washing hair, injudicious continuous bathing in river or pool and probing the ear with a stick or syringing of the ear. In most of the earaches, these come in late evening or at bedtime. The pains are sudden and acute and may or may not have redness or swelling of the ear passage.

First Step Treatment

- Never probe your ear with a stick to remove wax.

- If some foreign substance has entered the ear or there is hard wax, doctor has to be consulted to remove the same by syringing the ear with warm water.

- To remove that irritating wax, pour two to three drops of mullein oil (homoeopathic medicine) in the ears and plug them with cotton wool. Remove cotton plugs after 15 minutes.

- Do not put any other oil in the ears if there is pain or discharge from the ears.

- Cold currents of air should be avoided while you drive in a car or bike in winter. Wearing a helmet on bike or scooter is a good saver from earaches.

- In case of earache, hot fomentation is found of great help to mitigate the pain.

- Those prone to ear infections and pains frequently should plug their ears with cotton wool covered with petroleum jelly while swimming and taking bath. Better to avoid public swimming pools and polluted rivers or lakes.

Medicines

- Right ear: *Belladonna 30*, every two hours a dose, 5 doses a day.

- Left ear: *Chamomilla 30*, dose as above.

- Both ears: *Chamomilla 30* dose as above.

- Pain due to exposure to cold air: *Aconitum napellus 30*, dose as above.

- Pain extending to nose with frontal sinus: *Silicea terra 200*, one dose each for two days.

- Pain with sore throat: *Apis 30*, 5 doses a day.

- Repeated earaches: *Calcarea carbonica 200*, one dose each for two days.

- Tinkling, buzzing and stopping of ear: *Chamomilla 200*, one dose each for two days.

Fever Simple
KNOW ABOUT SIMPLE FEVER?

WHEN THE body temperature is above 37 degrees C or 98.4 degrees F, the condition of fever is stated. In other words, fever is abnormally raised temperature of the body. There is nothing to be worried about because it is an indication that some infection has entered the body and the immune system is fighting the infection to expel it. Fever is the result of this fight.

It is the mildest form of feverish attack and generally disappears in from twelve to thirty six hours. It starts mostly in afternoon or evening with alternating chill and flushes followed by heat and dryness of skin. The pulse is hard, quick, fast pulse rate, dry skin, dry coated tongue, thirst, scanty or coloured urine and anxious or rapid breathing. There may be pain in the body, headache, deranged bowels and loss of appetite. The cause is exposure to damp or cold, sudden change of temperature, poor or insufficient diet, fatigue, sore throat, internal or external injuries and viral infections etc.

First Step Treatment

- If the fever goes above 101 degree F, use cold, wet

compresses on the forehead, neck (back of), temples and wrists.

- Change the compress as it becomes hot until the temperature comes down.

- It is not advised to give a bath or cold sponge to the body with cold water because an abrupt drop of temperature may lead to shivering and it is not good for fever conditions/health.

- If it is summer, turn on the cooler or the fan and dress the patient in light comfortable clothes.

- Give the patient lot of fluids to drink so that patient passes lot of urine and has a sweating. Besides water, juice of lemon or orange (mausami) can be given.

- If the patient desires hot drink, give him tea with leaves of 'Tulsi'.

- Complete rest is best to fight fever infections.

- One should not feel hesitated to give allopathic drugs like 'crocin' or 'nimulid' when the fever has gone above 102° F and is not getting controlled by cold compress. These medicines will act as agents of lowering temperature and are not going to hamper the path of cure for homoeopathic remedies.

You need a medical help if:

1. The fever is high above 103 degrees F.

2. Fever does not come down even with cold compresses.

3. Fever is accompanied with severe headache or severe bouts of vomiting.

4. With fever, there is stiffness of neck, there is rash on the skin, there is severe abdominal pain, urine problems and total confusion.

F- 10

5. If it is an infant of the age of two to six months who has fever of 101 degree F or more.

6. A baby older than 6 months to one and half years has a fever of 102 degree F and above.

Medicines

❑   If the fever is due to exposure to cold winds and there is thirst, sweating and fear: *Aconitum napellus 30*, a dose every two and half-hours, total five times a day. Second day, give it four times a day and the third day onwards reduce it to three times a day. Give medicine for a total of six days.

❑   Face cold, hands warm, chilly, pain in abdomen: *Cina maritima 30*, four times on the first day and then three times a day for next five days.

❑   Fever with cough, aching of bones, thirst during chills, cough starts when chill starts, restlessness and diarrhoea may accompany fever: *Rhus toxicodendron 30*, in the above manner.

❑   High fever with tonsils-swollen, dry burning heat, red face, headache, feet icy cold, no thirst with fever: *Belladonna 30*, five times a day on the first day and on the second day, it is four times a day and rest of three days, it is three times a day.

❑   Fever with influenza, restlessness, drinks little water at a time but frequent thirst: *Arsenicum album 30*, four times a day on the first day and three times a day for rest five days.

❑   Fever with constipation, chilly and wants covering in the first stage of fever, chilliness when uncovered but still does not allow being covered, fever mostly starts in the morning: *Nux vomica 30*, same as above manner.

❑ First stage of all catarrhal and inflammatory fevers, headache better cold application, daily chill at 1 P.M.: *Ferrum phosphoricum 30*, four times a day the first day and three times a day for rest of five days.

Note : Do not give medicines when the fever is above 100° F and high. The best time for giving medicine is when the fever tends to come down.

Flatulence
KNOW ABOUT FLATULENCE?

FLATULENCE IS 'gas' in its simple definition. Local accumulation of gas inside the abdomen is flatulence. The gas moves about and may get expelled downwards (flatus), upward, or remain in the center of abdomen, distending it.

It is the most common disorder of the day to have flatulence or the wind in the digestive tract. In almost all cases, it is the result of constipation and indigestion but one cannot rule out possibility of irritable bowel syndrome, gallbladder stone and peptic ulcer. Gas starts with accumulation in abdomen that becomes bloated. This discomfort is relieved when the wind is expelled either through mouth or through anus. It is very much embarrassing and annoying when the gas releases out with a 'bang' in presence of others or when one has to cry out loud eructations.

First Step Treatment

● The best way to treat gas is to change your life style and eating habits. Adjusting diet will remove the problem by half if not more.

● Have a clear look at your menu and find out how much of fat and indigestible things are there. Over eating,

fatty, fried and fast food should be avoided. When food
is not digested and it is fermented, gas is produced.

- Taking of full pulses (Sabut Daal), beans, cabbage,
onions, carbonated drinks, uncooked food, unripe
fruits, food containing both starch and protein should
be avoided by those who are prone to flatulence.

- Do not take antibiotics without consulting the doctor.
Antibiotics change the metabolism and microorganism
of the intestines.

- Take light meals in the night and go for a walk.

- Get up early in the morning and hold a regular routine
of some light excercises.

Medicines

Only three first aid remedies are recommended:

◻ When the wind is locked up in the upper portion of
abdomen causing pain in the chest and difficulty in
breathing, eructations, heaviness, fullness and
sleepiness and abdomen greatly distended; better
passing wind: *Carbo vegetabilis 30*, four times a day
for two days. Reduce the dosage to three times a day
from third to sixth day.

◻ Gas with slight pain in the abdomen, weight in the
stomach after eating, takes more of tea and hence ill
effects of tea, belching of bitter fluid gives no relief to
gas, hiccoughs and gas is neither coming out from
mouth in the form of eructations or passing down from
the anus as flatus: *China officinalis 30* in the same
above manner.

◻ Gas due to taking fermented food, cabbage or beans,
excessive hunger, food tastes sour, eating a little creates

fullness, burning eructations rise to throat which burns for hours, abdomen is bloated and full: *Lycopodium 30*, three times a day for three days only.

Note : Consult a Homoepath after a week of taking above medicines when there is no relief.

Gum Disorders
KNOW ABOUT GUMS?

THE PLACE where your teeth rest firmly, the fitting area around the base of your teeth and the whole row of teeth, both upper and lower, make a continuous structure of flesh called gums. The good gracious gums need no geometrical explanations. Use the hard brush, get a blow on the jaws or try to pick-out trapped food particle, the gums will show their presence by bleeding. Apart from the injuries, if the gums bleed and are inflamed or cuase offensive odour in mouth is a warning that they need attention. Gum inflammation (Gingivitis) arises when plaque, a film of bacteria and residues of food developing on teeth daily, is not removed regularly by brushing and massaging. When plaque gets accumulated on the teeth and gum margins, it becomes a chalk like substance called tartar. Tartar in turn causes inflammation of gums. Ignoring the problem for long means depriving teeth of their security of gums. Teeth in turn will fall away and many serious problems of oral diseases may be experienced. This is one cause of inflammation or bleeding of gums, the other causes are poor nutrition and allergy to certain foods. If the oral hygiene including daily brushing and massaging with fingers is regular, the gum disorders are less by fifty percent. For detailed study of care of teeth and gums, read my book, 'Oral Diseases' published by M/s B.Jain Publishers, New Delhi.

First Step Treatment

• Brush your teeth daily in the morning with good herbal toothpaste.

- Before going to bed in the night, massage your gums and teeth with the help of herbal 'Manjan' (teeth cleaning powder).

- Make a weekly habit of using 'Datun'(thick twig of neem, margosa).

- After taking each meal, rinse your mouth with water for at least ten times.

- Do not take cold water immediately after taking hot food. Similarly do not take very hot things.

- Use a toothpick after each meal and rinse the teeth after it so that no particle of food is left in the teeth.

- In case of bleeding from the gums, apply mustard oil and salt on the teeth and gums with your fingers once a day. Leave the application for 10 minutes and spit. Do not rinse your mouth with water but go on spitting till you get the original taste of your mouth.

- Avoid sour things, onions, and red chilly and sweet foods.

- Chew your food properly and avoid constipation.

Medicines

- When there is bleeding while brushing, gums are swollen and thirst for very cold water, take *Phosphorus* 200, one dose and wait for three days to improve condition. In case of no benefit, consult a doctor. When the bleeding has stopped after taking *Phosphorus*, repeat one dose after ten days. If there is persistent bleeding after tooth extraction, one dose of *Phorphorus* 200 will stop it.

- When the gums are sensitive to cold air and water, there are boils on the gums, ulcerated and painful, take *Silicea terra* 200, one dose in the same fashion as above.

▫ When the gums are painful and there is soreness after tooth extraction, take *Arnica montana* 30, three times a day for three days.

▫ When teeth are sensitive and gums recede, blood comes out from gums when brushing teeth, take *Carbo vegetabilis* 30, three times a day for seven days.

▫ When gums are spongy, recede and bleed easily. There is sore pain on touching gums and pain from chewing, take *Mercurius solubilis,* three times a day for seven days.

Gallbladder Disease
KNOW ABOUT GALLBLADDER?

GALL IS bile and gallbladder is an organ attached to the liver storing bile. It is an important organ in our alimentary canal that helps in the process of digestion. Bile is a concentrated digestive juice produced by liver and stored in gallbladder. Gallbladder is stimulated whenever some fats enter the stomach or duodenum upon which bile is released from gall bladder and it breaks down fats for making digestion easy. If the stimulation of the gallbladder is less due to taking bland or infrequent food, the bile gets stagnant in the bladder and if this goes on frequently, chances of forming stone out of stagnant bile are more.

For complete details about gallbladder, please read my book,'Gallbladder stones and Kidney stones' published by M/s B.Jain Publishers, New Delhi. The prime disease of the gallbladder is development of stones in the gallbladder. Stones measuring upto two centimeters may develop or there may be smaller multiple stones. Many small stones develop and even pass out without knowledge of the person. Symptoms of pain come after the stones try to obstruct the passage or are too big and causing friction with the walls of gall bladder.

First Step Treatment

- Take less of non-vegetarian food (less of animal protein).

- Cut down your sugar and sweets intake.

- Cut down on starches and fats and calcium salts.

- Limit your intake of whole milk, cheese, butter, fatty things, cakes, biscuits and eggs.

- Take your food in time and do not delay for more than half an hour.

- Eat lot of vegetables and fruits like grapes, papaya, apple, coconut, mangoes and leechi.

- Avoid leafy vegetables and tomatoes.

- Take less of tea and avoid taking coffee.

Medicines (recommended as per P. 55 of my above-referred book on gallbladder stones)

- Dissolving or expulsion of stones: *Chelidonium majus-Q*, 10 drops in half cup of fresh water three times a day for 10 days. After 15 days, consult an experienced doctor, whose guidance is essential in the case of gallbladder stones.

- Colic: Take *Calcarea carbonica 30*, three doses at the interval of 10 minutes each. If the pain does not subside, consult a doctor.

- Preventing recurrence of forming stones: *China officinalis 200* every month one dose.

Note : For treatment of this disease, better consult a homoeopath than doing self medication.

Headaches
KNOW ABOUT HEADACHE ?

HEADACHE IS not an illness but a symptom of a general disease like indigestion, colds, flu, viral infection, lack of nutrients, sinus infection, excessive alcohol intake, fasting, dental problems, eye problems, hormonal changes and deranged menstruation and congestion and result of mental tension.

Pains can be mild, lasting only few minutes or prolonged. The headache may be in the form of heaviness, shooting from one point to another, fullness and heaviness in the eyes etc. It can be more with noise, light or mental efforts. The place of headache also differs. It may be on forehead, temples, above the head, back of head or sides of head.

First Step Treatment

- Take plenty of water.

- If you drink tea, there will be some relief.

- Massage the forehead and temples with oil.

- Apply pressure of fingers and fist over the painful area.

- Tie a cloth around head, if it soothes the pain.

- If you are a smoker, do not smoke when there is headache.

- Hot and cold compresses alternatively at the nape of neck will give relief.

You will need professional help if :

- Headache is from congestion or inflammation.

- Your headache has frequent and repeated occurence.

- There is stiffness of neck, vomiting, fever, skin rash and some problems in eyesight.

Medicines

- Headache with constant nausea, the tongue is clean: *Ipecacuanha* 30, three times a day for three days.

- Throbbing pain and heat felt in head during headache, pain is more on temples, forehead and occiput, pain worse from light, noises and lying down in the afternoon, rush of blood to head: *Belladonna*, six times a day for one day, four times a day the next day and three times a day for next two days.

- Due to over-eating, tongue white, headache worse bathing: *Antimonium crudum* 30, three times a day for seven days.

- Due to exposure to dry winds: *Aconitum napellus* 30, four times a day for one day, three times a day for next two days.

- Hammering type of headache, more when going in sun, during menses, headache of school- girls: *Natrium muriaticum* 30, three times a day for three days.

- Headache while studying: *Natrium carbonicum* 30, three times for seven days.

- Headache starts from nape of neck and shifts over to head, desire to lie quietly, better passing urine, headache from mental labour, smoking, and heat of sun: *Gelsemium sempervirens* 30, three times a day for three days.

- Bursting headache worst stooping, coughing and movement, more of thirst and constipation: *Bryonia alba* 30, three times a day for three days.

- Headache after grief, disappointment, death of a relative, inhaling smoke, headache worse stooping and as if nail was driven on sides of head: *Ignatia amra* 30, three times a day for three days.

- Headache due to sinusitis, pain at root of nose and

above eyebrows: *Kalium bichromicum* 200, one dose each for two days.

▫ Headache of women and girls due to eating rich fatty food, no thirst, headache better in open air, wandering pains in the head, pains starting from right temple region, headache from overwork: *Pulsatilla nigricans* 30, three times a day for seven days.

▫ Headache due to eye- strain, sewing work, pain as from nail and after excess of intoxicating drinks: *Ruta graveolens* 30, three times a day for seven days.

▫ Headache after taking alcoholic drinks, headache in the sunshine, sedentary habits, chilly patient, worse in the morning: *Nux vomica*, three times a day for seven days.

▫ Headache from sunstroke, or at menopause or due to suppressed menses. It decreases and increases with the sun: *Glonoinum* 30, three times a day for seven days.

▫ Headache begins from the occiput, spreads upwards and settles over the right eye and it is periodically say seventh day: *Sanguinaria canadensis* 30, three times a day for seven days.

▫ Pains below frontal eminence and temples and pain then extends to eyes. Feeling as if a band around the head. Headache starts from occiput and spread towards head and settles on left eye: *Spigelia anthelmia* 30, three times a day for seven days.

Hypertension or High Blood Pressure

KNOW ABOUT HIGH BLOOD PRESSURE?

WHEN THE circulating blood in the arteries creates a pressure on its walls and the pressure rises above normal, it is called high blood pressure. If we count reasons behind this disease, there are many from medical point of view but there are two main causes for a simple man to understand. They are lack of physical activity and stress or worries. If the style of living and thinking is changed, it will reduce high blood pressure. A normal pressure reading on the pressure- measuring instrument is 120/80 mm of Hg. Any reading more than 140/90 mm of Hg is high. The other reasons are obesity, excessive alcohol taking, sedentary life style, aging and some arterial diseases added by genetic factors. After the age of forty, one should get the blood pressure checked every month or so. The symptoms of high blood pressure are sometimes not well defined and there is not much of it felt by the patient until the pressure goes too high. Hence this check-up after the forty years of age is needed, especially for those whose parents have the same disease. During a check-up of some other disease or a routine medical check-up, if the blood pressure is found high even below the age of forty, this has to be taken care of. Smoking is also one of the causes of this disease.

Preventions

- Leave smoking, if you are a smoker.

- Try to conduct physical exercise daily, start regular morning walk, cycling or swimming.

- Have a diet free of fats and starch.

- Avoid taking excessive alcohol.

- Reduce your weight, if you are over weight by joining 'Yoga' classes.

- Reduce your intake of salt. There is a controversy over it although most of the doctors advice reduction in salt intake. Those persons who are sensitive to it only need reduction of salt. The best way to test the sensitivity is to reduce intake of salt for fifteen days. Get the blood pressure checked before and after starting this test to know the difference.

- Increase your intake of vegetables and fruits. Avoid non-vegetarian food.
- Take two pieces of garlic every day after breakfast.
- Try to avoid worries and stress in your job and business.

Medicines

First aid treatment: None at home. Better consult a doctor.

Note : No treatment suggested at home. Consult a doctor when you feel fainting, dizziness, tiredness and headache. If you have breathing difficulty, pain in the arms or chest and a sort of fear, consult a doctor immediately.

*Itching

Itching and Urticaria are different diseases and should not be confused with one another. Urticaria is itching due to prominent round or oval elongated patches of the skin just like nettle rash. These patches appear and disppear suddenly and are excited by scratching, exposure to cold and cause severe itch and heat.

KNOW ABOUT ITCHING?

ITCHING IS supposed to be both pleasant and troublesome. Its annoying and irritating character makes the person as if he/she is suffering from some serious skin disease. Itching may be due to a type of allergy, dryness of skin and irritation from certain perfumes, chemicals and household goods. Rich indigestible food, stimulating drinks, extreme hot and cold, a constitutional taint and chronic diseases are also responsible for itching. Those who have very sensitive skin are more prone to itching. Excessive bathing and washing of clothes with harsh soaps and detergents also cause itching. Sometimes itching may be on account of some thyroid problems or diabetes. Itching with eruptions is related to skin diseases while itching without any eruption may be due to allergy or mental stress.

First Step Treatment

• Whenever itching comes, better wet the place of itching by wrapping a wet cloth.

• Itching may be done, not by scratching the skin but pressing the area of itching.

• Minimising direct touch on the place of itching lessens it.

• Do not take a hot water bath. In most of cases, it increases itching.

• Do not use very strong smelling soaps for skin. Better use a mild soap or take a bath without any application of soap.

• If the skin is inflamed, it has eczema, it is infected or some underlying disease is the reason for itching, if the itching continues for a long time and if the patient is pregnant, consult a doctor.

Medicines

❑ Some parts of the body are so itchy that the patient draws out blood in his zeal for scratching: *Mezereum* 30, three times a day for three days.

❑ Itching without any eruption and the patient feels relief by rubbing the affected part against the wall: *Dolichos pruriens* 30, three times a day for three days.

❑ Itching in the bed and evening with dryness of skin, itching while undressing: *Sulphur 30*, twice daily for two days.

❑ When *Sulphur* has not worked, take *Carbo vegetabilis*

30, three times a day for two days.

▫ Itching with feverish feeling, redness of skin, thirst and itching more at night take: *Aconitum napellus* 30, three times a day for three days.

▫ Itching with redness, some swelling of skin and tingling, burning worse by warmth and eruption like urticaria: *Rhus toxicodendron* 30, three times a day for three days.

Indigestion
KNOW ABOUT INDIGESTION?

"DIGESTION IS a process where the food is taken in the stomach and other organs, for the formation of chyle, a milk like liquor, from which blood is formed for repairing the continued waste of the animal body. This process goes on in health easily, quickly and completely. Indigestion is a deviation from this healthy function in one or more of the qualities just named, it may be painful, slow or incomplete", says Dr. Ruddock.

The reasons for indigestion are eating too quickly, eating too much, changing to variety of foods, eating too frequently, eating fatty food and then eating fruits over it, drinking too much alcohol and tobacco, too many cold drinks, too much of tea or coffee, taking frequent drugs for indigestion without consulting doctor, smoking too much, eating fried, oily, heavy indigestible foods, eating at late hours, excessive body and mental strains. In a sum, taking things in 'too much' quantity is one of the main causes of indigestion.

First Step Treatment

• Persons with indigestion should correct all improper habits of eating as shown above.

• Do not eat too frequently.

- Do not eat too much of food.

- Chew the food properly. Proper mastication of food is a must. If you have some teeth problem like bleeding gums, carious teeth, decay etc., get it treated.

- Too great a variety of food at the same meal should be avoided.

- Take meals in time and do not take late dinners. Retire early and get up early.

- Do not take more than a glass of water during intake of meals. Water should be taken half an hour before or after taking of meals.

- Do not conduct exercises after taking meals.

Consult the doctor if:

- The attacks of indigestion are frequent.

- You are lacking in appetite day by day and your weight is getting less.

- The indigestion is experienced after the age of forty-five years.

- Self- medication has been done and this has increased your problems of indigestion.

- If you experience more of acidity when you wake up early in the morning.

- If the cough is also existing with indigestion for a long time.

Medicines

□ Acid dyspepsia- sour eructation, sour taste and vomiting: *Magnesium carbonicum* 30, three times a day for seven days.

- Dyspepsia of old, anaemic persons having heart burn: *Kalium carbonicum* 30, one dose each for two days.

- Indigestion of babies, overfed and intolerance of milk, vomiting curdled milk: *Aethusa cynapium* 30, three times a day for three days.

- With bitter, bad taste, after taking rich food, dislike for fats, thirstless: *Pulsatilla nigricans*, take in the same above manner.

- Chronic dyspepsia, aversion to food, hungry without appetite: *Cocculus indicus* in same above manner.

- Marked flatulence, belching after every meals, gastric ulcer, food intake brings pain in stomach: *Argentum nitricum* in the same above manner.

Insect Bites
KNOW ABOUT INSECT BITES

WHETHER YOU are living in a village or city, bites of insects like bee, wasp, mosquitoes cannot be avoided. Children playing in the gardens and play grounds covered with vegetation are more exposed to such bites. The pain, redness and swelling at the place of bite or sting is temporary but severe. Some people are sensitive to such bites and their skin reacts violently. Some get even fever after the bee or wasp bite. Mosquito bite may give rise to tiny wounds to some people. Mosquitoes puncture the skin whereas bee and wasp leave a sting in the skin.

First Step Treatment

- If it is mosquito bite, apply some smoothening lotion like calamine on the bitten area. To avoid itching, application of ice-cubes also helps.

- If it is bee or wasp bite, remove the sting by pressing it out from sides with the help of thumbnail.

- Still easier is to rub a piece of iron metal on the area of bee or wasp bite. Apply some lemon juice over it later and if this does not help, apply Urtica urens ointment or lotion.

Medicines

- For bites of bees: *Take Apis mellifica* 30, four times a day for one day.

- For bites of wasps: Take *Arnica montana* 30 in the same above order.

- For bites of mosquitoes: Take *Caladium seguinum* 30 in the above order.

Leucorrhoea
KNOW ABOUT LEUCORRHOEA?

LEUCORRHOEA IS a gynaecological problem. A discharge of various tints, usually white, occurs from inside the uterus or its covering and the os (mouth). Women and unhealthy young girls suffer from it and if neglected, the discharge becomes purulent and produces ulceration in and about the os. Headache, pale face, constipation, flatulence and dyspepsia are mostly associated with leucorrhoea. The causes of leucorrhoea are broken down health, chills, worms, dirt, stimulating food, excessive coitus, repeated abortions and irritation inside the uterus. In virgins, it is mostly associated with displacement of the uterus, congestion of the ovaries or general pelvic congestion and in married women, it may be connected with defective sexual hygiene.

When leucorrhoea is reported in children and young adults, it is usually confined to the vulva and vagina, rarely involving the uterus. The reason for little girls having this disease is measles and scarlet fever. The habit of masturbation may also be one of the causes in such cases.

First Step Treatment

- The hygiene of the patient must be carefully regulated.

- Digestion should be given special attention and tendency to constipation should be removed.

- Sexual hygiene has to be taken care of. Excessive and frequent indulgence in sex should be avoided.

Medicines

□ Acrid and watery: *Natrium muriaticum* 30, three times a day for seven days.

□ Profuse, making parts raw : *Acidum fluoricum* 30 in the above manner.

□ Profuse, dark, bloody: *Agaricus muscarius* 30 in the above manner.

□ Leucorrhoea instead of menses: *China officinalis* 30, in the same manner.

□ Nursing women leucorrhoea: *Acidum phosphoricum* 30 in the same manner.

□ Chronic with pain and lameness in back, dark yellow, thick: *Aesculus hippocastanum* 30, in the same manner.

□ Discharge leaves yellow stains on clothes: *Chelidonium majus* 30 in the same manner.

□ Acrid, yellow discharge, low backache, worse between periods and after periods: *Kreosotum* 30 in the same manner.

□ Acrid, curd like or white of an egg like with warm sensation of flow: *Borax veneanta* 30 in the same manner.

□ With backache: *Ova tosta 3x*, in the same manner.

- Green or yellow with acrid discharge, constipation, bearing down sensation, before periods and leucorrhoea of little girls: *Sepia officinalis* 30, in the same manner.

- Milky, creamy, loss of thirst, emotional women: *Pulstatilla nigricans* 30, in the same manner.

- Burning, itching more at night: *Mercurius solubilis* 30, in the same manner.

- Burning itching, milk like, before and after menses, in little girls : *Calcarea carbonica* 30, in the same manner.

- Acrid, ropy, stringy, profuse, transparent, running down to heels, worse day time, after menses, better by washing: *Alumina 30*, in the same manner.

- Profuse, white, itching and constipated, in fat obese females, during menses: *Graphites* 30, three times a day for 5 days.

- Purulent, gushing between menses, extreme weakness, nausea during journeys: *Cocculus indicus* 30, three times a day for 7 days.

Important Note : In case of no relief, treatment after seven days should be under guidance of doctor. In case of relief, no repetition is needed. Wait for 15 days and then take one dose of the same medicine in 200 potency. Watch the results. Relief means no further medicine.

Menses Problems
KNOW ABOUT MENSES OR MENSTRUAL PROBLEMS?

MENSES IS an indication that the sexual life of woman has started. Once every 28 days, a woman passes blood from her genitals for 4 successive days. Every woman differs from these norms. The age of puberty, the age of menopause, the duration of menstrual period all differ. Menses is usually associated with the bursting of an ovum in the ovaries and renewing of the uterine endometrium. Conception has no relation to menses, it can occur independently of menstruation. The sensitive balance of hormones in the monthly menstrual cycle can change by various factors like change in thermal environment, weight of body, diet, exercise and stress or worries. There are many problems associated with the cycle. The menses may be painful, heavy, irregular, infrequent and scanty.

Pain during the periods is very common ailment for little girls, teenagers and young women. This problem mostly gets over after marriage, childbirth, or after the age of twenty five or so. The pain is felt in the lower abdomen like cramps with discomfort or pain in the back and sometimes nausea is also there.

Irregular menses is due to irregular ovulation and it occurs during the first few years after the first menses. It is again irregular when the menopause approaches.

Heavy periods is mostly in the beginning of menses and then in late thirties or forties and the cause is hormonal disbalance, stress, change in diet or pelvic inflammatory diseases, fibroids or endometriosis.

Scanty periods may be due to anaemic conditions, hormonal disbalance, taking contraceptive pills, weight loss and eating disorders.

Pregnancy during the periods generally does not occur but it is possible in some cases. It is always better to use a reliable method of birth control during intercourse. Intercourse during menses is not prohibited medically. It is a decision between the husband and wife's comfort. For exercise during menses, there is no prohibition. Light exercises should be preferred.

First Step Treatment

Before one week of the onset of menses,
following is recommended:

- Take extra care to have a healthy diet, which should

have essential fatty acids, vitamin B, C and E, calcium and magnesium.

● Vegetarian food, lot of green vegetables, plenty of fluids and fruits should be taken.

● Proper measures should be taken that constipation does not exist.

● Avoid stimulants like coffee, tea and alcoholic drinks.

● Conduct regular exercise like brisk walking, swimming, joining Yoga classes.

● Do not take extreme hot and cold things and avoid extreme temperatures of climate.

Medicines

Note : No medicine should be given during menstruation. Better give after the cessation of periods or at least 8 days before menses.

Menstrual Pains relief

❑ Violent pains associated with heat and bright red, clotted blood: *Belladonna* 30, six times a day for a day.

❑ If pain is shooting and there is less of pain with gentle massage on the abdomen and hot compress: *Magnesium phosphoricum 6x*, 4 tablets six times a day with lukewarm water.

❑ If pain is relieved by doubling up and by warmth, take *Colocynthis 30*, four times a day for one day.

❑ A warm bath or heating pads relieve the mild pains.

❑ Conduct some light exercise like brisk walking or swimming, cycling or jogging. It is useful only for some women.

Excessive Menses (Menorrhagia)

□   Pain in the back down thighs and through the hips with heavy pressing down. Severe pain all through the flow. More of flow, more of pain: *Cimicifuga racemose* 30, three times a day for seven days.

□   Excessive flow with same above conditions but lasting long with dropsy (swelling of body) and change of life: *Apocynum cannabinum* 30 in the above manner.

□   Excessive and early with headache, colic, chill, leucorrhoea before menses, burning and itching of parts before and after menses, anaemia and vertigo: *Calcarea carbonica* 30 in the above manner.

□   Excessive and early with abdominal distention: *Nux vomica* in the same above manner.

□   Excessive, early, intermittent, during night and lying down: *Kreosotum* 30 in the above manner.

□   Excessive, early by two weeks or so, worse after exertion: *Medorrhinum* 200, one dose for a day.

□   Excessive, clotted, offensive, difficult to wash, due to fibroid: *Platinum metallicum* 30, three doses for seven days.

□   Excessive continued to next period, dark, clotted, irregular: *Secale cornutum* 30 in the above manner.

□   Excessive, acrid, frequent, after miscarriage: *China officinalis 30* in the same above manner.

□   Excessive, dark, frequent, irregular, offensive, during day-time only : *Lilium tigrinum* 30 in the above manner.

□   Excessive, late, or suppressed, worse sitting, better after flow starts: *Zincum metallicum* 30 in the above manner.

□ Excessive on alternate periods, painful, first day scanty, second day with vomiting: *Cyclamen Europaeum* 30 in the above manner.

Scanty Menses

□ Menses, scanty, short, difficult and late, thick black acrid flow: *Sulphur* 200 one dose for one day only.

□ Menses scanty, spasms accompanied by vomiting: *Cuprum metallicum* 30, three doses a day for seven days.

□ Menses scanty for one day only with pain in stomach and back during periods: *Baryta carbonica* 30, in the above manner.

□ Menses scanty with weeping tendency and irregular, painful, consolation aggravates: *Natrium muriaticum* 30 in the above manner.

□ Scanty, painful, increases while sitting, less while walking: *Alumina* 30, in the same above manner.

Early Menses

□ Early and prolonged for 7 to 10 days with leucorrhoea like white of an egg before menses, pains and thirst is less: *Gelsemium sempervirens* 30, three times a day for seven days.

□ *Calcarea phosphorica* 30 (puberty and wetting feet during menses) and *Nux vomica 30* (black blood with fainting spells) can also be given when symptoms are same as in *Gelsemium sempervirens*.

□ Early, prolonged with terrible itching, left leg becomes blue and painful, aggravation lying down, discharge of blood between periods on accidents: *Ambra grisea* 30, three times a day for seven days.

- Early and profuse, with bearing down, debility: *Sepia officinalis* 30 in the above manner.

- Early, profuse, suppressed after bathing in swimming pool, tongue white coated: *Antimonium crudum* 30 in the above manner.

- Early, profuse with thick and strong odour, offensive: *Carbo vegetabilis* 30 in the above manner.

Late, Suppressed Menses

- Menses late, scanty and suppressed: *Pulsatilla nigricans* 30, three doses a day for seven days. If it fails, follow it up with *Sulphur 200*, one dose for a day and then on the third day after giving *Sulphur*, give *Pulsatilla nigricans* again for seven days.

- Late, scanty, suppressed due to cold or wetting hands, breasts become large, sore: *Conium maculatum* 30, three doses a day for seven days.

- Late, scanty with extreme weakness: *Sepia officinalis* 30, three doses a day for seven days.

- Menses, late, scanty, painful lasting for one hour or one day only with ophthalmia (eye problems): *Euphrasia officinalis* 30 in the above manner.

- Delayed, especially first menses,painful, scanty, constipated: *Graphites* 30, three doses a day for seven days.

- Menses not starting at puberty: *Lycopodium clavatum* 200, one dose weekly for three weeks and then consult a doctor, if it does not come.

- Menses late starting in girls, dark blood: *Ferrum metallicum* 30, three times a day for seven days.

- Menses suppressed in girls for months: *Sabina 30*, in the same above manner. If it fails, consult a doctor.

Menopause Problems
KNOW ABOUT MENOPAUSE?

BY THE time, a woman is 40 to 45 years of age; menses tend to stop. This is the stage called menopause. When menses stop, a woman's capacity to bear children comes to an end. A new phase of life starts, which brings lot of changes. Menopause is, therefore, called change of life too. This transition brings in physical changes with mental and emotional problems. Some women nurture a wrong idea that they are not fit for any sexual enjoyment in absence of menses. They feel guilty on this account and the result is number of psychological and physical diseases. There is no timing for menopause to begin and it depends upon the life style, diet, tensions, worries and medication. There is a reduced production of hormones by the ovaries and supply of oestrogen hormone falls when approaching menopause. It falls rapidly afterwards and comes to stabilizing level. The first symptoms of menopause are hot flushes and night sweats and these symptoms continue for months and even years. Pain is felt during intercourse due to dryness of vagina. Headache, sleeplessness and tiredness with depression are other symptoms.

First Step Treatment

• Start regular exercise, long walks and other physical activities like swimming, dancing etc.

• Pay more of attention to your health and well being than caring or worrying for other members of family.

• Take plenty of vegetables and fruits.

• Light nourishing diet, excellent and cheerful surroundings, fresh air and gentle exercises are required.

Note : If there are sudden changes in mental or physical conditions, a doctor has to be consulted.

Medicines

❑ Take *Lachesis mutus* 200, one dose every fifteen days. Two doses for a month only if you have hot flushes, night sweats, bleeding heavy, cramps in uterus, burning sensation in head, aggravation of symptoms after waking and more of irritability.

❑ Take *Sepia officinalis* 200, in the same above manner for one month if alongwith hot flushes and night sweats, there is pain in vagina during sex. Lot of weakness is felt after doing little work.

❑ Take *Pulsatilla nigricans* 200, in the same above manner when you have a weeping tendency due to the menopause, mentally irritable, hot flushes, swinging of moods and emotions to bad and good, changeable behaviour with members of family and less of thirst for water.

Migraine
KNOW ABOUT MIGRAINE?

MIGRAINE IS paroxysmal headache. Headache is severe, recurrent and intense ; commencing mostly in the morning and which may be unilateral, frontal, occipital or general. It may last for two to three days in mild form and brings lot of weakness. The headache has a long years of standing from childhood and sometimes it is in the later years of life. It may be associated with vomiting and hence called sick headache, or bilious attacks. There may be peculiar disturbances of vision also in some cases.

First Step Treatment: None

Preventives

● One should know from which condition, circumstances and eatables, the headache commences. There may be certain allergic foods. Make a note of food you had taken before the onset of headache to check it next time.

● Get your blood pressure checked and if it is low, get its treatment.

● If you have some mental worries and tensions, find out a solution.

● If you are not getting enough of sleep, have a check up with doctor.

● If some bright lights in the room or extremely noisy music upset and trigger your headache, make arrangements to avoid it.

● If the headache comes in certain climate or change of season, talk with your doctor about it.

● If the headache is due to onset of menopause or due to hormonal changes, the treatment is different and help of doctor is needed.

Medicines

▫ From worries, excessive studying by students and teachers, pains on right side, burning of stomach and bile vomiting, attacks come in hot weather or change of weather: *Iris* 30, four times a day for two days and three times a day for two days.

▫ Right sided pain above eyes, periodical headache, say, every eight days, early morning and on rising: *Sanguinaria canadensis* 30, three times a day for four days.

▫ From mental work, cold, uncovering head, pressure, sun heat: *Glonoinum* 30, three times a day for three days.

▫ From abuse of alcohol, coffee, spices, tobacco. Late night sleeping, worry, sexual excesses, head congested: *Nux vomica* 30, four times a day for three days.

▫ From disturbance in menses, climacteric changes, women having different moods in a day, weak and having yellow spots on nose or cheeks. The pain is mostly on left temple: *Sepia officinalis* 30, four times a day for two days and three times a day for another two days.

▫ From excessive noises, loud music and change of weather. Pale face and pain is sharp on the left side of face and left eye. Pain may travel from occiput to left eye. Vomiting is associated when pain is more or at height. Pain more in the morning and it improves when the sun sets: *Spigelia anthelamia* 30, three times a day for three days.

▫ From the onset of menopause or before menses, pains worse during and after sleep, it is left sided: *Lachesis mutus* 200, one dose only.

Mouth Ulcers
KNOW ABOUT MOUTH ULCERS?

MOUTH ULCERS are small, white or yellow ugly looking eruption occurring in the mouth cavity.

Ulcer may be single or in clusters on tongue, beneath tongue, inside the cheeks, on the palate or behind lips. They are very painful. The reason is underlying infection, digestive upset, wrong type of diet, stress, wrong fitting of new denture, injury by a biting of tongue, allergy of some particular food item or food sensitivity. Mouth ulcers known as aphthous ulcers or stomatitis are very painful. They have a white floor and yellow border, small and superficial, they have tendency to recur and heal up within seven to fourteen days. (For detailed knowledge, read my book, 'Oral Diseases' published by M/s B.Jain Publishers, New Delhi).

First Step Treatment

● Do not take much of sweets and starch.

- Avoid very hot drinks and meals.

- Wash out oral cavity with water after every meal. Brushing of teeth also helps.

- Avoid use of more of salt, lime and mercury (in drugs).

- Nutrition in diet has to be maintained.

- For infants, keep the feeding bottles and spoons clean and sterilized after every feed.

- Child should not be given dirty toys to play with. The toys should be washed and cleaned.

- Leave smoking and chewing tobacco.

Medicines

▫ Small ulcers of aphthous type, they bleed when touched, mouth feels hot and tender: *Borax veneta* 30, four times a day for two days and three times a day for next two days.

▫ Salivation is more, the gums are bleeding and are spongy, taste of mouth is metallic and there is thirst although the mouth is moist: *Mercurius solubilis* 30, three times a day for three days.

▫ Mouth ulcers with sharp splinter like pain, salivation is offensive and acrid, the ulcers are more of red in appearance than white: *Acidum nitricum* 30, three times a day for three days.

▫ Mouth ulcers of any type but there is headache also accompanying ulcers: *Belladonna* 30, four times a day for two days.

▫ Mouth ulcers look like blisters, they are sensitive to touch and one feels better if he holds cold water in the mouth: *Natrium sulphricum* 30, three times a day for three days.

Note :

- If the ulcers are due to new denture or caused due to old denture, consult a dentist.

- If the mouth ulcers are recurring, it is better to consult a homoeopath.

- If the healing does not take place within 15 days inspite of homoeopathic or allopathic treatment, better consult a specialist of oral diseases.

Neck Pain, Cervical Spondylosis
KNOW ABOUT NECK PAIN?

STIFFNESS AND pain in the neck is a common disorder of the day. This condition involves muscle pain in the area surrounding neck and cervical region, morning stiffness and immobility of the muscles of neck. The reasons are too much of exercise, lifting heavy weight, wrong sitting and standing postures, exposure to cold air, sleeping on an elevated pillow and soft mattress, insufficient nutrients, cramps, fatigue, tension, stress, anxiety and depression.

Muscles pain may also be a result of injury on the neck area. Cervical spondylosis is a condition pertaining to degenerative process caused by degeneration of the intervertebral discs with the formation of bony ridges running across the anterior surface of the neural canal and also due to the formation of osteophytes from the neurocentral joints of Luscka, which project backwards into the intervertebral foramen. For complete detailed study of cervical spondylosis, please read my book, 'Neck Pain-cervical Spondylosis' published by M/s B. Jain Publishers, New Delhi).

Five Points to Identify Your Neck Problems

- Mobility is the first thing that reminds that there is something wrong in the neck.

- The second thing is pain in the neck and adjoining area.

- The third thing is persistent aching or stiffness along the spine from the base of neck.

- The fourth thing is sharp localized pain in the neck radiating to either the shoulders or hands or the upper back.

- The fifth thing is that there is chronic ache in the neck area if it is not cared with.

First Step Treatment

- Avoid faulty postures in sitting, standing, reading, writing and doing work on computers.

- Avoid mental stress and worries.

- Avoid sleeping with head on highly elevated pillows.

- Avoid muscle fatigue by not driving the car or scooter too long a distance.

- Avoid holding the head in one particular position over a long period as in the case of viewing cinema, driving cars etc.

- Take plenty of rest. Rest means immobilization of the affected part. This should be only limited to the extent that the neck pain is relieved. Excessive rest is not required.

- When sleeping, remove the pillow from beneath your head and lie on a hard bed.

- A hot compress is usually helpful to remove pain in the neck. Electric heat pads, hot water bottles or hot packs made of folded soft cotton cloth may be used.

- Regular exercise of the neck is needed. Forward and backward, side -wise and circular movements of neck, clockwise and anticlockwise, are beneficial when there is no neck pain.

• 'Yogasans' are also quite useful for neck pains and this should be done under the guidance of an expert.

• Massage of neck by palms lubricated with mustard oil also helps remove pains.

Medicines

▫ Neck stiffness after overuse as in driving, viewing cinema. The pain reduces with gentle movement and aggravates when lying down: *Rhus toxicodendron* 30, four times a day for three days.

▫ Neck stiffness and pain when exposed to dry cold winds and pain is more when neck is moved, thirst is also more with pain: *Bryonia alba* 30, four times a day for three days.

▫ Neck pain due to exercises, falls, and bruises, sleeping on too hard a bed with head on elevated pillow. The pain is more when moving the neck: *Arnica montana* 30, four times a day for three days.

▫ Sudden pain in neck after exposure to dry cold winds, pain is worse at night and on moving the neck, restlessness and thirst is more: *Aconitum napellus* 30, four times a day for two days and three times a day for one day.

▫ Pains are not stationed on neck but go on shifting to fingers, wrists, hands, lower spine when sitting and pains are more in cold air: *Kalium bichromicum* 30, four times a day for three days.

▫ Pain in large muscles of the trunk, spinal nerves and cervical. Suited to women who suffer from uterine and ovarian affections. Pain comes suddenly like electric shocks. Pains are sharp, lancinating with a feeling of stiffness and retraction. The pain also wanders around the neck but prefers left side of neck in most cases. Pain worse at night, motion, cold and during menses:

Cimicifuga racemosa 30, four times a day for three days. Do not take any medicine during menstruation. Consult a homoeopath.

❑   When neck pains are shifting from one side to another and patient has vertigo. The severe pains are mostly on right side of neck and there is numbness too. The pains shift downwards and the shifting is rapid. Pains worse by motion, exertion and open air, looking down and bending forward: *Kalmia latifolia* 30, four times a day for three days.

Numbness
KNOW ABOUT NUMBNESS?

A **FEELING,** in any part of the body as if there is no sensation, is called numbness. In general terms, it is called sleeping of limbs and one experiences it when sitting in one posture for a long time. The cause of numbness is feeble circulation of blood, tensions, indigestion, constipation and heart ailment.

First Step Treatment

●   Jerk the limb getting numb and if this does not help, give a gentle massage.

●   Take a cup of tea without milk mixed with four to six drops of lemon juice.

●   Take a cup of milk without sugar mixed with two teaspoonful of 'Isabgol'.

●   If you have started exercises and jogging recently and having numbness as a consequence, stop exercise and resume after advise from doctor.

●   If there is numbness in head, consult a doctor.

Medicines

▫ Feet, fingers and soles, staggering, cannot pick small objects, sleeping of limbs: *Alumina* 200 one dose at night for three days.

▫ Head numbness with pain: *Asafoetida* 30, three times a day for three days.

▫ Back and limbs numb, swelling of ball of thumb: *Oxalicum acidum* 30, three times a day for three days.

▫ Dead feeling, parts cold and blue: *Agaricus muscarius* 30, three times a day for three days.

▫ Hands and fingers numb in the morning and during night, worse heat and sleep: *Lachesis mutus* 200 one dose weekly for two weeks.

▫ Forearm numb at night: *Argentum nitricum* 200, one dose at night for three nights.

▫ Limbs go to sleep on slight pressure, lying down, feeble circulation: *Ambra grisea* 30, three times a day for three days.

▫ Numbness of any part of body but with pain: *Chamomilla* 30, three times a day for three days.

Nails, Affections of
KNOW ABOUT NAILS DISORDERS?

NAILS ARE said to be in healthy condition when they look smooth, strong and have colour of flesh, somewhat pink. If nails have grooves, lines, rough looking, spoon shaped and getting broken easily, they are unhealthy. Some doctors see the condition of nails and judge the condition of your health. The reason behind this logic is that the nails are made of keratin, a type of protein, which is the main content of skin and hair. If protein is less, the body reflects. If a nail is removed or broken due to some injury, it takes about six months to grow from base to tip. A toe nail may take more than six months to grow. White spots on some nails do not indicate any disease but some doctors view it as deficiency of zinc in the body. Of course, iron-deficient nail can result the profile of each nail to become spoon-shaped. Iron deficiency or anaemia changes the colour of nail to pale and make it brittle. Huge deficiency of protein in the body can make a nail bed appear white. If bacteria infect the nails and its surrounding skin, nails can become soft, discoloured and thick. Some skin diseases also make the nails look dirty, damaged and thick.

First Step Treatment

- As soon as you notice a change in nail's condition and colour or the nails are growing late or too soon, consult a doctor.

- Cut your nails regularly so that there is no dirt in them.

- After washing the hands and feet, dry them thoroughly.

- Wearing of gloves while washing utensils or clothes is a good care for nails.

- Take care of your diet. Have key-nutrients like items containing calcium, vitamin C and zinc.

Medicines

The medicines given here should not be expected to fetch immediate results. It is a slow process just like growing of nails and hence patience is needed. After first self- medication, Homoeopath has to be consulted.

- Corrugated and spotted, uneven and rough nails: *Calcarea carbonica* 200, one dose daily for four days. Watch the results after 15 days and consult homoeopath.

- Thick, brittle, black and easily falling nails, constipation and pain in back: *Graphites* 200, one dose on alternate nights for three nights. Consult doctor after 15 days.

- Nails grow too fast, deformed, uneven, break easily and are brittle: *Acidum fluoricum* 30, three times a day for seven days and then wait for one more week before reporting to doctor.

- Waxy, distorted, soft and brittle nails, sweating on covered parts of the body, patient goes for stool after taking breakfast: *Thuja occidentalis* 200, one dose daily in the night for four days. Report the result after 15 days to the homoeopath.

- Discoloured and distorted nails, likes salt very much: *Natrium muriaticum* 200 in the above manner as written against *Thuja ocidentalis*.

- Loose, painful, sensitive nails, even pains when cutting nails: *Hepar sulphur* 30, three times a day for five days. Report to doctor after fifteen days.

- Root of nails painful: *Calcarea phosphorica* 30, three times a day for seven days.

- Nails grow slowly: *Causticum* 200, one dose a day for three days. Watch for fifteen days and report to doctor.

- White spots on nails, nails look crippled, ingrowing toe nails, affection on the surrounding skin of finger nails: *Silicea terra* 30, three times a day for seven days. Result may be watched for two weeks and reported to homoeopath.

Nausea (Vomiting)
KNOW ABOUT NAUSEA OR VOMITING?

NAUSEA IS sickness or disgusting feeling of vomiting. Vomiting is actually throwing up the contents of stomach. Everyone has these two symptoms at one time or the other. Both nausea and vomiting are mostly due to digestive problems, taking too much food or taking such food to which one is allergic, intolerent or sensitive. These symptoms are also produced by taking too much alcohol, some toxic substances (food poisoning) or by some infection. Migraine or headache, motion sickness such as traveling in vehicles and fear/anxiety can also cause vomiting. Nausea also occurs in pregnant women, and children get vomiting due to high fever in some cases. Some allopathic drugs also induce nausea for some persons. A stomach ulcer and gall bladder stones can also cause vomiting.

First Step Treatment

- Give the patient lemon juice in water or 'Pudin Hara' or some digestive 'churan', or ginger tea available in Indian homes. They help reduce the preliminary nausea and vomiting.

- Take care of kitchen hygiene and avoid taking one type of food that triggers vomiting.

- Instead of taking heavy meals, take frequent light meals.

- While eating, maintain a habit to eat slowly. Do not be in a hurry.

Medicines

- The first important remedy is *Ipecacuanha* 30 in all types of vomiting. Give a dose after vomiting every time the patient vomits. After the first dose itself the vomiting will stop.

- In case of nausea, give *Ipecacuanha* 30 one dose and wait. If the vomiting occurs, give another dose after vomiting.

- For journey sickness and vomiting, give *Cocculus indicus* 30, half an hour prior to start of journey and then one dose in the vehicle when the patient feels nausea or one dose after the vomiting.

- For vomiting of pregnant women, give a dose of *Sepia officinalis* 30 after vomiting. Do not repeat. If the complaint persists, better consult homoeopath

- When you feel like vomiting and think that vomiting will be better to ease your stomach problem, take a dose of *Nux vomica* 200.

- When there is gastrointestinal problem and diarrhoea with occasional vomiting, burning of stomach, weariness and chilly feeling, take *Arsenicum album* 30, four times a day for two days.

Nose Bleeding
KNOW ABOUT NOSE BLEEDING

IN COUNTRY like India where the hot climate brings many diseases, nose bleeding is one of them found mostly in children. Adults do not have nosebleed. Old people may have it in some cases. The reason is rupture of small blood vessels of nasal lining either due to heat or frequent nose boring / pricking with fingers and even due to heavy sneezing. This disorder is almost insignificant and can be handled at home. If the nose bleeding is reccurring in adults or old people, they should contact the doctor for blood pressure checking and blood clotting disorders. This is very rare. Please note that we are not talking about Epistaxis ('Naksir' in Hindi).

First Step Treatment

- Press and pinch your nostrils with thumb and index finger while you lean a little forward in sitting position. Keep the head upright. The practice of tilting the head backwards and pinching the nose may also stop bleeding but there is a chance of flow of blood from head to throat and this may choke you sometimes. A child gets the choking due to tilting of head. Keep the pressure on the nose for 15 minutes.

- Release the pressure of fingers and if bleeding is still not stopping, keep it pressed in the same manner for another ten minutes.

- Even if the bleeding does not stop, make a mixture of cold water and alum. Wet a cloth in this mixture and keep the wet cloth on the forehead for some time. Tell the patient to lie down when putting cloth on forehead.

- Applying ice pack on the nose also stops bleeding.

- After the bleeding stops, take a cup of lukewarm milk and a banana.

Note : If the nose bleed is due to some injury on head, if the bleeding lasts for more than fifteen minutes inspite of above measures and taking homoeopathic medicines, if the bleeding from nose is a frequent occurence and if the loss of blood is more, contact a doctor immediately.

Medicines

□ *Ferrum phosphoricum* 30 should be given, three doses, one after the other at the interval of 5 minutes. If the bleeding stops after one dose, do not repeat the medicine.

□ If the bleeding is sudden and very heavy, a dose of *Phosphorus* 200 will stop bleeding.

Obesity or Overweight
KNOW ABOUT OBESITY?

THE BEAUTY of the body lies in its appearance. A dynamic personality and a towering appearance are all gifted from the parents (genetic make up) but the upkeep of body lies with the individual. If one allows the body to grow fat by dint of sedentary habits and excessive fats taking, it has to look fat or obese. So, more than the limit of fat in a body with reference to the height of the body is injurious for health and such a condition is called obesity or overweight. Obesity, therefore, occurs due to more food intake and less calories burnt. Now many schools conducting 'Yoga' and aerobic exercise alongwith the control of diet are attracting obese persons to control weight. As a matter of fact, medicines act less than the measures one takes to cut the body weight. Overweight increases the risk of serious illnesses like heart diseases, hypertension, diabetes, digestive problems, osteoarthiritis, infertility, varicose veins, menstrual problems and pregnancy problems.

First Step Treatment

Those who are prone to gaining weight should take following steps :

- The food should be taken in time.

- While breakfast and lunch may be taken as usual, the dinner may be taken very light.

- Chew the food properly and never in a hurry.

- Avoid taking more of sugar and sweets, more of fats and fried things.

- Take a plate full of seasonal 'salad' before the meals.

- Take at least two or three glasses of lukewarm water in a day.

- Take regular exercise or join a 'Yoga' class.

- Change your eating habits in consultation with 'Yoga' or aerobic exercise teacher.

- Do not go for crash diet programme, which helps loose weight only for a short while. Excessive weight loss is through sensible and healthy eating.

- There are many health clubs or companies, which assure reduction of weight within a very short time. These are very expensive programmes and may have side effects too, because they give drugs suppressing appetite. This will affect digestion and absorption of food. Even if medicines are to be preferred, better to go in for safest homoeopathy.

How do you know that you are overweight?

First of all, you will yourself say that you are overweight. Your figure will tell that. Secondly your friends and relatives will declare that you have put on weight. And finally it is you who has to check it either with the doctor or carry out following tests at home by yourself.

The thumb rule is that if your body weight is 20% more than its normal value for your height, you will be called obease. The best method to know about your overweight is to know your body mass index or BMI. BMI is calculation of your height and weight. The other method is to know the ratio of your hip and waist measurements. It is here that most of the fat accumulates.

KNOW YOUR BMI

1. Divide your weight in kilograms by the square of your height in metres. Suppose your weight is 68 kilograms and height is 1.50 metres, the BMI will be 30.22, which will be called obese. (68 divided by 2.25 i.e. square of 1.50).

2. BMI under 20 is underweight.

3. BMI from 20 to 25 is healthy.

4. BMI 26-29 shows overweight.

5. 30 or more means you are obese.

Another rough rule to know about
the overweight is as follows:

If the body weight is 50 kilogrames, it is normal weight for a person of five feet height. On an inch above five feet, add 2 kilogram to 50. This means that a person of five feet one inch height should have normal weight of 52 kg. Five feet two inches will have a normal weight of 54 Kg. You can make plus or minus two kg. in the arrived figures. This means that a person of 5 feet height having 50 to 52 kg. of weight is normal. (5 feet is 1˙.52 metres)

Please note that above method is only a rough guidance for body weight in adults (Men and Women) based upon average calculations. Here is a chart for some measurements:

Height		Weight acceptable range in kg	Obese in kg	Grossly in kg
In mt	In feet-inches			
1.45	4-9	42-53	63	84
1.48	4.10	44-55	66	88
1.50	4.11	45-56	68	90
1.52	5.0	46-58	69	92
1.54 to	1.66 (i.e. 5-1 to 5.5)—Go on adding two kg in above figures.			
1.68	5.6	56-71	85	113
1.70 to	1.80 (5-7 to 5-11)—Go on adding two kg in above figures.			
1.82	6.0	66-83	99	132

And so on as per above rule of adding two kg.

Medicines

◻ Medicines can only help you reduce the weight only when you are taking regular exercise and improved diet as per recommendations given above. If the diet and exercise reduces your weight by one kg a month, medicine alongwith the restrictions of diet and exercise will reduce the weight by two kg a month.

▫ 10 to 15 drops of *Phytolacca berry -Q* should be taken three times a day preferably 15 minutes before each meal for one month. Upon finding a weight loss, further medicine be taken on advise of homoeopath.

▫ If obesity is due to thyroid problems, take *Thyroidinum* 200, weekly one dose for a month and consult the doctor afterwards.

▫ If obesity is due to goiter or thyroid enlargement and patient has constipation and flatulence problems, *Fucus vesicatoria -Q* should be taken as per dose and frequency shown against *Phytolacca* above.

Note : There are many patent homoeopathic medicines named differently claiming trim and slim figure after their uses and are easily available in the market. They are mixtures of homoeopathic medicines like Phytolacca berry, Fucus vesicatoria, Thyroidinum, Ammonium bromatum, Calcarea carbonica, Pulsatilla nigricans, Silicea, Antimonium crudum, Graphites and so on. I have no comments upon their utility because I do not believe in mixtures at present.

Operation After-effects
KNOW ABOUT AFTER EFFECTS OF
. SURGICAL OPERATIONS

A SIMPLE cut on skin while shaving or cutting vegetables has after effects, if the injury is not cared for. If someone undergoes a surgical operation-involving cutting of skin, there are bound to be after effects for which antibiotics are usually given to heal the wounds. When the operation is performed by a surgeon of the conventional system of medicine, there is no fun of refusing to take the medicine prescribed by the surgeon, if healing is the motive.

Homoeopathy has additional benefit of healing the after effects of operations in shorter time (Removing gall bladder or uterus, kidney stones, hernia or appendix operations or even complicated heart bypass surgery).

First Step Treatment : None

Medicines

- *Rhus toxicodendron* 30 is general medicine for all after effects of operation. 4 pills three times a day for 10 days after the operation.

- For restoration of damaged nerve tissues: *Hypericum perforatum* 30, in the above manner.

- When damage to intercostal nerves and muscles is involved in operation: *Cimicifuga racemosa* 30 in the above manner.

- When there is injury to nerves in the extremities during operation: *Hypericum perforatum* 30 in the same above manner.

- When damage to nerves is on the left side of the body: *Spigelia anthelmia* 30 in the above manner.

- Pain in nerves in fractures and stumps due to operations: *Symphytum officinale* 30 in the same above manner.

Opposite Symptoms and Remedies
KNOW ABOUT OPPOSITE SYMPTOMS?

HERE IS a wonderful example of finding a remedy when two organs of the body or two opposite symptoms are found in one disease. As a first aid method, the medicine so prescribed in opposite symptoms gives relief in most of the cases. For example if cough aggravates during inhaling, one remedy is given but if the cough aggravates during expiration, the remedy is different. Inspiration and expiration the process of respiration are examples of opposite symptoms.

First Step Treatment : None
Medicines

□　Cough aggravates on expiration: *Aconitum napellus* 30, three times a day for seven days.

□　Cough aggravates on inspiration: *Spongia tosta* 30, in the same manner.

□　Cough aggravates going from warm to cold air: *Phosphorus* 200, one dose only, watch for the results upto four days.

□　Cough aggravates going from open air to warm room: *Bryonia alba* 30, three times a day for four days.

□　The edges of tooth decay: *Mercurius solubilis* 30, three times a day before sunset for four days.

□　The roots of tooth decay: *Mezereum* 30, in the same above manner.

□　Dry mouth without thirst in any main disease/ disorder (It is unusal symptom because when the mouth feels dry, there is desire for water, here it is different): *Pulsatilla nigricans* 30, three times a day for five days.

□　Moist mouth with thirst in any main disease/disorder: *Mercurius solubilis* 30, three times day before sunset for five days.

□　Diseases (for example headache) begin on left and then go to right side: *Lachesis mutus* 200, one dose and wait for results upto four days.

□　Diseases begin on right and then go to left side:

Lycopodium clavatum 200, one dose and wait for results upto a week.

□ Acrid (irritating) coryza (cold) with bland (non-irritating) lachrymation (tears): *Allium cepa* 30, four times a day for four days.

□ Acrid lachrymation with bland coryza: *Euphrasia officinalis* 30 in the same above manner.

□ Toothache ameliorates by heat or hot food or tea etc.: *Magnesium phosphoricum* 30, four times a day for four days.

□ Toothache ameliorates by cold water, ice cream: *Coffea cruda* 30 in the same above manner.

□ Colic (Pains) ameliorates from bending the body double: *Colocynthis* 30, four times a day for three days.

□ Colic ameliorates on bending backwards: *Dioscorea villosa* 30 in the same above manner.

□ Sweats as soon as one closes his eyes to sleep: *Conium maculatum* 30, three times a day for three days.

□ Sweats when one wakes up: *Sambucus nigra* 30, three times a day for three days.

□ Constipation before and during menses: *Silicea terra* 30, three times a day to be taken one week before the expected date of menstruation. The medicine is not to be taken during menses.

□ Diarrhoea before and during menses: *Bovista lycoperdon* 30 in the same above manner.

□ Child is good and playing whole of the day but restless, screaming and trouble whole of night: *Jalapa 30*, two times a day for a week.

□ Child cries whole day but sleeps well whole of night: *Lycopodium clavatum* 200, one dose for one week.

Piles (Haemorrhoids)
KNOW ABOUT PILES?

PILES ARE small tumours outside or inside the opening of the lower bowel either with or without bleeding. Numbers of such tumours also vary. It may be a single intensely painful swelling or a number clustering together like a bunch of grapes. These swellings are painful, itching, pricking, shooting and throbbing, burning or pressive and the pains increase on going to stool and sometimes with dull pains in the loins. Blood oozes out like a stream in alarming quantity with every attempt of passing stool and at times, the blood comes only by drops after or in mid of passing stool. The cause is constipation, a long standing obstinate constipation not cared for in the past, taking purgatives and continuous intake of hard indigestible, fried and stimulating rich spicy food. The sedentary habits and a luxurious life is also another reason. Excessive excercises, horse riding, sitting on cold stones, damp grass and pressure of enlarged womb upon the vessels of the pelvis during pregnancy are some other causes of piles.

First Step Treatment

- Avoid spices, alcoholic beverages, indigestible foods, and coffee, fried and fatty food.

- Take properly cooked vegetables and ripe fruits and avoid non-vegetarian food.

- Too much standing, sedentary habits, use of cushions and very soft bed should be avoided.

- In blind piles (no bleeding) the pains can be removed by frequent washing of the anus with cold water or tepid water (whichever is found agreeable). One should sit in the tub of cold or tepid water for some time or a wet compress be applied as soon as the piles are starting to pain.

- In bleeding piles, the pains are less but can be removed

by drinking a glass of cold water and taking rest (lying down) for one hour.

● After every evacuation, ten to fifteen minutes of lying down gives relief to the pains.

Medicines

Piles–Bleeding

❑ When the blood is bright red, give *Millefolium Q*, ten to fifteen drops five times a day for two days. Reduce the frequency on the third and fourth day when bleeding stops.

❑ When the blood is dark clotted, the evacuation is with soreness and pulsating pain, give *Hamamelis virginiana-Q* in the above manner.

❑ When the bleeding is in a small stream alongwith every evacuation, give *Phosphorus* 200, one dose after stool. If the bleeding stops in next evacuation, no medicine needed and if the bleeding occurs again, give another dose but in no case, more than two doses of *Phosphorus* should be given.

❑ When bleeding is accompanied with constipation or diarrhoea alternating with constipation and there is loss of appetite and bleeding is painful, give *Collinsonia canadensis-Q*, in the same manner as in the case of *Hamamelis*.

❑ When there is bleeding with cutting pains for hours after passing stools, give *Acidum nitricum* 30, four times a day, preferably after evacuations.

❑ When the piles are bleeding or non-bleeding but occurring only during climacteric (menopause), give *Aesculus hippocastanum* 30, four times a day for three days.

Note : When the bleeding does not stop after two days of medications as above, consult the homoeopath.

Piles - Blind

□ When there is pain in lumbo-sacral region and anus feels as if full of sticks, give *Aesculus hippocastanum* 30, four times a day for three days.

□ When haemorrhoids look like onions and are purplish in colour with hammering and throbbing in anus, give *Lachesis mutus* 200 one dose every day in the morning for three days.

□ When the urge is there to pass stool frequently, there is constipation also with itching and stitching after eating, when mental exertion is also a cause, give *Nux vomica* 30, four times a day for three days.

□ When there is biting sensation and soreness in anus, anus is moist due to constant oozing, give *Paeonia officinalis* 30 in the same above manner.

□ When there is protrusion of anus after every stool, give *Podophyllum peltatum* 30 in the above manner.

□ When there are cracks and deep fissures in anus, there is pain after passing stool and patient is restless, the orifice of anus is constricted, give *Ratanhia peruviana* 30 in the same above manner.

□ When the haemorrhoids protude like bunches of grapes after every stool and application of cold water relieves, give *Aloes* 30 in the same above manner.

□ When the stool is mixed with mucous, pain during evacuation and the tongue is white coated, give *Antimonium crudum 30* in the above manner.

□ When the pains are of burning nature and washing anus

with cold water does not relieve pain but with lukewater water or warm applications if the pain relieves, give *Arsenicum album 30* in the same above manner.

▫ When even walking is painful due to piles, give *Causticum* 30 in the same above manner.

▫ When the pain has sensation as if red-hot iron is thrushed into rectum and pain is better by applying cold water, give *Kalium carbonicum* 30, three times a day for one day only.

▫ When there is swelling and protrusion of piles, blind or bleeding, the stools are not constipated but much of flatulence, skin is sensitive to touch and even contact of cloth is intolerable, give *Acidum muriaticum* 30, four times a day for three days.

▫ When Piles come out every time patient urinates, there is constipation with hard knotty stools and a sensation of crawling in the rectum, give *Baryta carbonica* 30 three times a day for four days.

Prostate Gland Disease
KNOW ABOUT PROSTATE GLAND?

PROSTATE GLAND is the property of men. Women do not have it. It is situated just below the bladder and is normally of the size of walnut. The job of the gland is to secrete a fluid, which is said to enable the sperm to swim and reach woman's cervix at the time of ejaculation. The diseases or problems come up when the gland becomes inflamed or enlarged. It then obstructs the passage of urine (urethra) complicating the micturition (act of urination). This gland is also a general place for cancer in old men. The problems generally begin after the age of fifty years when the prostate starts to get enlarged. This condition does not call for any treatment till there is obstruction in urine flow. This also can result in frequent urge to urinate and the patient goes for urination frequently but the flow is very slow or drop-by-drop. The urine passes in small amounts and takes lot of time. Inflammation of the prostate gland is called prostatitis and may occur due to excessive sexual acts transmitting infections or doing some exercises while the urinary bladder is full. In prostatitis, there may be backache, abdominal pain and fever and pain while urinating. In case of cancer of prostate gland, there are no symptoms and only periodical blood tests after the age of forty can detect cancer. According to some medical experts, there will be some sort of uneasiness during coition accompanied by some pains in the scrotum area.

First Step Treatment

- If you have difficulty in urination as per symptoms stated above, consult a doctor.

- Take lot of leafy vegetables and simple food containing fibres so that you are not having constipation.

- Drink two glasses of water in the morning on empty stomach.

- Do not retain your urine for a longer time when there is urge for urination. Go for its call.

- Do not conduct exercise when your bladder is full and you feel like urinating.

- Before taking a bath and after taking meals, go for urination. Make it a habit.

- Avoid unprotected sexual acts.

- Avoid smoking and excessive intake of alcohol.

Medicines

- Inflammation and enlargement of prostate gland, take *Sabal serrulata-Q*, 10 to 15 drops in half cup of water three times a day for 15 days and report to homoeopath. It is head remedy and can be continued for a longer time till homoeopath advises.

❏ When the urine stops and starts, the patient can pass urine only when standing and he or she is old bachelor or widower, give *Conium maculatum* 30, three times a day for seven days.

❏ When the patient dwells on sexual objects, has urge for urine but when passes it dribbles in small quantity, give *Staphysagria 200*, one dose daily at bedtime for four days.

❏ When the patient is old and has childish behaviour, he or she is shy to tell symptoms, give *Baryta carbonica* 200 in the above manner.

❏ In old persons, when there is pain during the act of urination, frequent micturition at night with a full feeling of pressure in the rectum and at times, retention of urine too, give *Ferrum picricum-30*, four times a day for seven days.

❏ When the urge for urination is more and frequent pressing to pass, strains much to pass but passes little urine, give *Thuja occidentalis* 30, three times a day for seven days.

Sore Throat
KNOW ABOUT SORE THROAT?

SORE THROAT is pain in the throat area. Generally, sore throat is considered to be the first symptom of incoming cold, throat infection, glandular fever or flu. The sore throat is due to some allergy, cold dry air, pollution of atmosphere, and viral or bacterial infection. If the sore throat is not accompanied with any cough, fever, or coryza, it is managed by gargles with warm salt-water or black tea with salt. Taking a cup of hot water with salt in it in the fashion as you take tea, also helps remove throat pains. This should be done at least two times a day.

First Step Treatment

- It is better to gargle the throat as suggested above for at least four to five times a day.

- Keep the throat wrapped with warm clothing, if it is winter.

- Avoid smoking.

- Avoid going to a crowded area where pollution is more.

- Take plenty of rest for a day.

- Gargle your throat with 10 drops of *Phytolacca decandra Q* mixed in 100 ml. of luke warm water. This may be done two to three times a day. It gives good result in all the cases of sore throat.

Medicines

- Sudden pain in throat area due to exposure to dry cold wind and patient is worried: *Aconitum napellus* 30, four times a day for three days.

- The throat is burning, dryness of throat, unquenchable thirst but takes water little at a time, give *Arsenicum album* 30, three times a day for three days.

- Pain in throat, which is worse by empty swallowing, patient can swallow liquids comfortably but not solids, tonsils are swollen, give *Baryta carbonica* 30, three times a day for four days.

- Throat is painful and appears red hot, pain is due to congestion. Throat also swollen with burning and the pain is on the right side of throat: *Belladonna* 30, four times a day for three days.

▫ Throat appears to have pus formation, shooting and piercing pain, throat sensitive to cold and touch, patient is chilly but perspires, give *Hepar sulphur 30*, three times a day for four days.

▫ Throat pain on left side and then it shifts to right side, it has purple colour inflammation, even pressure of clothes around throat is intolerable, give *Lachesis mutus* 200 one dose in the morning for one day and watch. If needed give another dose on third day.

▫ Throat and tonsils pain starting from right and then shifting to left, the nose is stopped, give *Lycopodium mutus* 200 one dose in the above manner.

▫ When throat pain is shifting from any one side to other side frequently, give *Lac caninum* 30, three times a day for three days.

Snoring
KNOW ABOUT SNORING?

SLEEPING AND snoring are made for each other. Snoring comes after sleep and does not disturb the snoring- person. It disturbs the sleep of others, who toss, turn and get tortured nights after nights. Medical science has made tremendous progress and conquered over many diseases but to abate snore is a distant dream. Why to blame scientists, even public is not serious to have it cured. People consider it a disorder and not disease. Snoring has gained international fame because of its menace of sleeplessness for the room partners, who in turn do not hesitate to seek divorce on this account. The characteristic feature of snoring is that snoring persons do not agree that they snore during sleep. A noisy breathing during sleep is snoring. Rattling noise during inspiration, produced by vocal cords or by vibratory action of the pendulous palate during sleep is snoring. If there is narrow nasal passage due to polyp, chronic atrophic rhinitis, chronic rhinitis, acrid, and corroding catarrh, a person breathes through mouth. This is snoring. If the pillow used is old, broken, causing discomfort and is too low, the mouth gets opened and the noise thus produced is snoring.

First Step Treatment

- Try to reduce your weight.

- Avoid smoking and alcoholic drinks.

- Use a pillow a little higher, say about 8 to 10 centimetres from bed.

- Use nasal clips or strips, which are meant to help easy breathing and available in the market.

When to consult the doctor?

When you snore loudly and often; when you wake up and feel tired; when you choke or hold your breath during sleep; when you often feel sleepy during waking hours and when you are overweight or your neck is thick, it is better to consult the doctor.

Medicines

- When the snoring is due to obstruction of nose and enlargement of nasal bones, give *Lemna minor* 30, two times a day for 15 days.

- When there are caries or enlargement of nasal bones with swelling and redness of nose and obstinate catarrh, give *Hippozaeninum* 30 in the same above manner.

- When it is a child who has blocked nose and has sleep apnoea with cough and snores, give *Sambucus nigra* 30, three times a day for seven days.

❑ One dose of *Bacillinum 200* given at the interval of 15 days, two doses in a month is helpful in removing snoring habit. It should be given and progress be watched after a month. In between the period of no medicine, give *Silicea terra* 12 X for one month except on the day, *Bacillinum* is given. *Silicea terra* 12 X should be given three times a day and one dose is 4 tablets.

Styes (Eruption on the Margin of Eyes)
KNOW ABOUT STYES?

A BOIL like eruption, nodule or a small abscess in the eyelid, normally at the base of eyelash of either lid or corner of eyes is called a stye. Styes are most of the times frequently occurring in some persons. They are painful and with swelling. A tired eye exposed to pollution, smoke and dust make the eye infected. The reason of stye is still unknown but it is known that it is not a serious disease. There is an old saying that the stye occurs to those persons who continuously and frequently look at their stools, while evacuating. Another saying states that styes are due to over-indulgence in sex (newly married couples or otherwise). There is no scientific proving to these causes but it is not going to harm anyone if he or she does not look too much at the stools and avoids excessive sexual acts. Old sayings are sometimes very useful hints of health.

First Step Treatment

● It takes about a week or so for a stye to recede or vanish of its own, even if it is not treated. The styes mostly burst releasing the pus or heal by disappearing very slowly.

- Styes are supposed to be contagious and hence separate towels and handkerchiefs should be used.

- There should be frequent washing of face and hands.

- Try not to touch eyes or styes.

- Do not try to squeeze the stye so as to take out pus.

- It will burst of its own and then do wipe the area carefully so that the pus does not touch the inner surface of eye.

Medicines

▫ For chronic or recurring styes, mostly on the lower lids, or on either of lids of children, give *Staphysagria* 200, two doses at the interval of three days.

▫ Styes mostly on the upper lids but can be on either lids and when the patient is fond of taking fats, rich and greasy food, give *Pulsatilla nigricans* 200, in the same above manner. *Pulsatilla nigricans* should be the first choice.

▫ Styes recurring and itching as well on the margin of lids, give *Silicea terra* 200 in the same above manner when *Pulsatilla nigricans* has failed.

Toothache
KNOW ABOUT TOOTHACHE?

TOOTHACHE IS pain in the teeth, which is a result of a decay or abscess or inflammation inside the tooth or of the gums. Most of the time, the people opt for treatment from a dentist but there are number of home treatments and homoeopathic application for simple toothaches to relieve the pains. Tooth decay is the result of accumulation of plaque, a film of food residues or saliva or even bacteria. This plaque absorbs starch and sugar from the food particles and produce acid that can destroy the enamel (the protective surface of the tooth). If precaution is taken by cleaning the teeth by brushing after each meal or after taking sweets/starch, the risk of pain in teeth is reduced. If the acid is not removed and it remains on the tooth, it penetrates and forms a cavity allowing bacteria enter the pulp within the tooth, painful abscess cannot be ruled out. (For full details on the upkeep and care of teeth, read my book, 'Oral Diseases' published by M/s B.Jain Publishers, New Delhi).

First Step Treatment

- Clean the teeth twice a day, early in the morning and before going to bed.

- After taking each meal, rinse your mouth with water for at least ten times.

- Do not take cold water immediately after taking hot substance.

- Do not take very hot or very cold things.

- Use a soft toothpick after each meal and rinse the mouth after cleaning.

- Avoid taking pickles, when the toothache has started. Pickles have acidic nature and may weaken the enamel.

- Calcium, vitamin C and D are necessary for dental health. Take lemon, carrot, radish, 'Amla', groundnut, butter, milk, honey, curd, orange, banana, coconut and mangoes from time to time, season-wise in moderate quantity.

- Do not take 'Gutkha', chew tobacco or smoke.

- Take tea at least twice in a day. It has fluoride that

fights tooth decay.

● Do not take much of carbohydrates like white flour (Maida) and sugar in excessive quantity. It will add to plaque formation and raise acid level in the mouth.

● Let dentist examine your teeth at least once or twice in a year.

Medicines

External application

▫ When the tooth is painful, *Plantago major-Q or Echinacea angustifolia -Q* may be applied with the help of cotton wool ball. This will reduce the pain.

Rub some drops of clove oil on the gums above or beneath the painful tooth for many times till the pain gets less.

Internal

▫ When holding cold water in the mouth relieves toothache, pain worse at night, more of thirst and more of saliva in mouth: *Mercurius solubilis* 30, three times a day before sunset for three days.

▫ Toothache is better when holding ice cold water in mouth: *Coffea cruda* 30 in the same above manner.

▫ When drinking cold water and even hot tea aggravates toothache, give *Mercurius solubilis* 30, two times a day and *Sulphur* 30 one dose in the morning for five days.

▫ Under the same above condition, if the above foes not relieve after three days, give *Mercurius solubilis* 30 two times a day and *Aurum metallicum* two times a day in alternating fashion for three days.

▫ Pain extending to ears and teeth feel elongated: *Plantago major* 30 in the same above manner.

▫ Pain worse by pressure and decay is in the roots, mastication gives pain and teeth are sensitive to touch and cold water, pain extending to eyes also: *Staphysagria* 30 in the same above manner.

▫ Shifting of pains from one tooth to other with swelling of face, pain better by heat and hot drinks: *Kreosotum* 30 in the same above manner.

▫ Warm water increases pain, pain radiating to ears and face: *Chamomilla* 30 in the same above manner.

▫ Inflammation of decayed tooth, worse night, cold or hot application: *Mercurius solubilis* 30, three times a day, take it before sun set.

▫ Pain in hollow teeth worse by eating, drinking cold water, night: *Antimonium crudum* 30 three times a day for three days.

▫ Pain worse taking anything sweet: *Natrium carbonicum* 30, in the same above manner.

▫ Pain worse after loss of vital fluids in the body: *China officinalis* 30 in the same above manner.

▫ Pain due to pyorrhea and gums swollen: *carbo vegetabilis* 30 in the same above manner.

▫ Pains after extraction of teeth, bleeding from teeth after filling in cavity: *Arnica montana* 30 in the same above manner.

▫ Throbbing pains scattered all around mouth, dry mouth and gumboil: *Belladonna* 30, four times a day for three days.

▫ Pain even on slightest touching of the teeth and they bleed easily, worse in cold air: *Hepar sulphur* 30 three times a day for three days.

U.T.I.
(Urine Tract Infection)
KNOW ABOUT UTI?

THE INFECTION or inflammation of lower part of urinary tract, which is urethra and bladder, is UTI. It is mostly seen women. Short urethra in women permits easy infection. The symptoms are pain, burning or scalding during urination. There will be frequent and sudden urge to urinate and some pain is also felt in lower abdomen. Urine may turn milky (pus contents) or bloody and even smell badly. In acute cases, fever may accompany. This is no serious disease but if it is neglected and not taken care of through medicines and alternative methods, the kidneys can get damaged. Bacteria usually cause the infection. It is mostly found in large intestine and can easily travel from intestines to the anus and then to urethral opening and upwards to bladder. When it is not cured, bacteria settle in the bladder lining and causes inflammation. Further deterioration can affect kidneys.

First Step Treatment

- Take plenty of water to flush out bacteria.

- Stop taking hard drinks, coffee, alcohol and stop smoking.

- Wash the genital with water after each act of urination. This should be done even when there is no urineary infection.

- Wash the genital area before and after the intercourse.

- While washing the anus after stooling, take care not to wipe anus in the direction towards genital. Wash and wipe it in the opposite direction so that bacteria in stool do not travel to urethra.

- Make sure that you change sanitary napkins frequently.

- Do not wear tight underwears.

Medicines

▫ When the urine is burning, painful and it is frequent but when passing it appears hard to pass, emission drop by drop: *Cantharis vesicatoria* 30 four times a day for four days.

▫ When the burning exists while urinating and last drops of urine are most painful, there is no thirst and patient is restless: *Apis mellifica* 30 in the same above manner.

▫ When the burning of urine is there and the pains are at the conclusion or end of urination: *Sarsaparilla officinalis* 30, four times a day in the above manner.

Voice-Disorder
KNOW ABOUT VOICE DISORDER OR

Voice Loss?

VOICE DISORDER or loss of voice is very common in India where marriage functions, public meetings and teaching contribute a lot to it. In marriage and other functions, people talk and sing, in public meetings, leaders talk loudly for hours and in schools, teachers have to speak continuously in their classes. Voice loss is due to disorder of vocal cords and it affects the normal speech. Either the voice becomes harsh or less audible or even lost. The loss is temporary and it is due to inflammation of the larynx (voice box). The other reason is viral infection due to cold, smoking and taking irritating foodstuff. If the voice loss is a regular feature and persists in some persons, it may be due to polyps (benign growth on the vocal cords). This needs a medical check up by a doctor. If the voice loss is due to excessive use of voice as in leaders, speakers and teachers, it goes of its own within few days. The inflammation or infection, in such cases, is painless.

First Step Treatment

● Rest to the larynx and avoiding overuse of the voice will bring speedy cure.

● Do not clear your throat frequently as it may lead to irritation of larynx.

● If you had cold and after it, there is voice loss or hoarseness, treat the cold first.

● Take plenty of water.

● Giving steam to the throat and gargles with black tea mixed with some salt for three to four times helps a lot.

Medicines

□ Loss of voice from cold or simple catarrh: *Causticum* 30, five times a day for two days.

□ Loss of voice when exposed to severe heat: *Antimonium crudum* 30, four times a day for two days.

□ Sudden loss of voice of singers, public speakers or lawyers: *Arum triphyllum* 30, five times a day for two days.

□ Loss of voice before menstrual period: *Gelsemium sempervirens* 30, four times a day for two days before onset of periods. No medicines during periods.

□ Voice changes in tone and sometimes it is uncertain or like whispers: *Rhus toxicodendron* 30, four times a day for two days.

❏   Any type of voice loss or hoarseness with thirst for very
    cold water: *Phosphorus* 200 two doses in all at the
    interval of one hour.

Varicose Veins

KNOW ABOUT VARICOSE VEINS?

WHEN THE veins on the body are swollen or twisted and are
painful, such a condition is called varicose veins. High pressure
inside veins damages their valves and result in blocking of blood.
This build up of blood makes veins swollen and become like
knots or twisted. Such a condition can be anywhere in the body
but most affected parts are legs. In a leg vein, valves stop blood
from going down the leg due to gravity. When these valves are
not functioning properly, the blood collects there and dilates the
veins. They turn blue and lumps appear. This condition is found
in the backside of leg i.e. calves or inside of the legs. In some
cases, the pain is severe and swelling even travels to ankles.
The discoloration also occurs in some cases due to
eczema/ulcer formation. The only treatment in the conventional
system of medicine is operation but changing of life style and
diet alongwith use of homoeopathic medicine can bring some
relief.

First Step Treatment

●   Make it a habit to go for a walk at least after dinner and
    early in the morning. This will improve the circulation
    of blood in the legs.

●   If you are overweight, try to reduce the weight.

●   Do not stand for a long time or sit still for a long
    period.

●   When sitting try to put your feet up on a stool. Do not
    put a stool beneath your calves, which will obstruct

blood supply.

- Those who have a job requiring long standing (doctors and nurses in operation theatre) should go on shifting their body weight from one leg to other.

- Whenever you return from work, lie down for some time with legs raised above the level of your head. For this remove the pillow from your head and place two pillows beneath legs.

- In air journeys or long railway journeys, better move around for ten to fifteen minutes every one or two hours.

Diet and Yoga

- Diet plays a useful role in curing varicosity of veins. Switch over to vegetarian food immediately if you are non-vegetarian. Take plenty of vegetables and fruits. All citrus fruits can be taken because of their quality of containing nutrients to make veins strong and elastic. Vitamin C is helpful in this respect. Fibre rich food should be taken so that there is no constipation.

- Yoga is a wonderful healer of varicose veins. 'Sarvang-asana' (standing on shoulders) and other associated 'Asanas' are very useful. For complete set of exercises in Yoga, consult a Yoga expert.

Medicines

External application

□ In all types of varicose veins, apply lotion of *Hamamelis virginiana* twice a day, after bath and at bedtime.

- Varicose veins with purple areola and veins are blue or purple: *Aesculus hippocastanum* 200 two times a day for 7 days and then consult a homoeopath for further treatment.

- If varicose veins are on left leg and are blue or distended: *Ambra grisea* 30, three times a day for 7 days and then consult a doctor.

- Severe pain in legs and patient is unable to move even: *Hamamelis virginiana* 30 in the same above manner.

- Varicose veins with ulceration: *Acid fluoric* 30 in the same above manner.

- When the patient tries to keep legs elevated because bringing them down makes him feel that the legs would burst: *Vipera aspis* 30 in the same above manner.

- If the varicose veins have appeared during pregnancy, take *Pulsatilla nigricans* 30 in the same above manner.

Note : It is always better to consult a homoeopath for curing this disease.

Warts
KNOW ABOUT WARTS?

WART IS a small, circumscribed epidermal and papillary elevation of the skin, which is also called verruca. There are many types of warts for which different remedies are given according to their location, symptoms and shape. Warts are called innocent growths and it is oftenly removed for cosmetic reasons in conventional system of medicine. Children and young adults are more commonly affected. They are due to microorganisms and are feebly autoinoculable and contagious. However senile warts are due to nutritional changes in the skin, incident to old age, while venereal warts are by contact with a local irritating secretion which may contain a causal germ. In general we can say that warts are contagious growths of dead skin cells and they remain on the outer layer of skin. In children and young adults, most of the warts disappear from six months to two years. There is no treatment except surgical removal in conventional system of medicine but homoeopathy has remedies for it.

First Step Treatment : None

Medicines

◻ When warts are like cauliflower, in crops, are moist and bleed easily on touching: *Thuja occidentalis* 1 M, one dose weekly for three weeks.

◻ When warts are solid, horny type or flat on face, neck area, tip of nose and on fingers: *Causticum* 1 M, one dose weekly for three weeks.

◻ When warts are itching, bleed easily, soft, spongy and having stinging sensation: *Calcarea carbonica* 1 M, one dose weekly for two weeks.

◻ When warts are on back of hands, large, fleshy or smooth on hands and face: *Dulcamara* 1 M, one dose weekly for three weeks.

◻ When warts are on palms and painful or on soles (corns) with yellow colour: *Ferrum picricum* 30, three times a day for two weeks.

◻ When warts are pendunculated type, bleed easily, painful, and large: *Acidum nitricum* 1 M, weekly one dose for three weeks.

Note : It is better if a homoeopath is consulted after the above treatment even if there is improvement with these medicines.

Tips for success

IF YOU are a BHMS student, if you have finished your studies and started practice, if you are a person who has interest in homoeopathy, you must have felt that whenever you have given some medicine to a patient and the patient is cured, you get an inner happiness. If this happiness is limited to your mind and it has not gone to your head, it is healthy thinking but if this happiness is mixed with pride and you get bloated with feeling of abundance of knowledge, you are not going to achieve high goals in homoeopathy. The success must be taken as granted if your knowledge is more than sixty percent in the subject and failure should be taken as a lesson that you need more of studies. Do not get worried and try to find out the actual reason of your failure in prescribing the remedy. Success should be pondered over as to how success was achieved and how it could be made more fluent. Failure should be taken as a challenge to probe the weakness in selection of the remedy. This is one aspect of thinking about success and failure.

DISEASE IN MIND

One must agree that all diseases in the body or mind are due to a denied feeling behind it. Great Dr. Hahnemann has given high importance to mind but think of our ancient Indian philosophy. It is far beyond the thinking of philosophers of other countries. Our great cultural, social and scientific upgradation has no match. The calculations made on distance of planets in the universe without adequate scientific gadgets (astrology and astronomy described by 'Aryabhat') makes the world wonder about the wisdom, Indians possessed. Similar is the case in the field of medicines.

In our ancient books of medicines, we predicted much before great Hahnemann about the super powers of mind.

Here are some surprising facts. Try to verify by yourself practically and you will find them at least seventy five percent true. Probably, I found them in that percentage but you may find them absolutely true.

- If you have fear, rage, worry or sadness stored in your body and you have not been able to tell it to your beloved ones or near-dears, you are likely to get a cold.

- If the grief and sadness has been stored in your body for a very long time and you are not exposing it to others, you are likely to get cancerous tumors in the long run.

- If you are not in the habit of showing your anger or rage in the childhood due to your attitudes or fear of elders and this trend of suppressing anger is carried over to adulthood, you are likely to get arthiritis.

- If you had great sexual desires in the childhood and carried over to adulthood, if the same desires were not fulfilled due to late marriage and if married in time but the sexual satisfaction was not in accordance with the fantasies, you are likely to get skin diseases and asthma.

SUCCESS LIES IN PERSONALITY

The most important factor in achieving success is not known to you but your patients know it. Is it not surprising?

- The personality in a doctor is not the figure, well built body, proportionate structure, fair complexion, beautiful or handsome features and charming personality.

- The personality of a doctor lies in his/her way of dealing with the patients, giving a keen careful listening to the patients, talking pleasing words of assurance of health restoration and appreciating the interests of the patients.

- Instead that the patient wishes the doctor, 'good morning' etc., if doctor wishes the patient first, it adds charm to the personality of doctor.

- The doctor's personality is always under vigorous vigil by the patients. If the doctor is short, bald, bespectled, dark and not pleasing to look at, it makes no difference with the patient. It is the glare of health that beams out of doctor's face that attracts the patients.

- If the doctor is sick, wiping his red nose, coughing frequently, having fluent coryza and looks pale, patients feel sicker. 'An ailing person can not cure others' is the general thinking of patients. Whenever you are not well, better absent yourself from the clinic.

- If the doctor has a thick appearance of having burden of domestic worries or tensions, if he or she appears to have vibrations of anger, sadness, fear or rage on his/her face, it will be easily read by the patients. They would not like the very idea of getting in touch with unacceptable feelings that turn off their belief that a doctor is a person who showers happiness. Try to wear a happy and smiling face and this will be additional charm to your personality.

- Keep in mind that secret of a healthy body is not your medicines given to your patients. It is above type of personality and convincing power that works more than your medicine.

- The secret to a healthy body is a healthy mind, a mind that is free of stress and negative thoughts.

- The patient coming to you needs your sympathy and assurance in such a way that his/her mind and soul feels hopeful of a recovery.

Your patients will return to you a number of times with different disorders when they find that your behaviour towards them is friendly and that you give them the best of attention. This is the exact personality, a doctor should possess.

LUST FOR MONEY : BIGGEST FOE

If you are a BHMS student or completed the studies and practicing, your worries are money- earning and competition in the market. As a matter of fact, you entered this profession with a given understanding that it will offer you very good money. Right from the childhood, every one of us has been fed with the idea that money is the real source of joy and that you have to work hard to get money. Money is not the source of joy; this can be evidenced from very rich people. They are not happy and always burdened with worries. The second aspect that money can be earned only by hard work is true. Have belief in this saying and work hard to survive. Your ego will make sure that you work hard. On the other hand, if you go on worrying that patients are very less and what will your parents or friends think about you, you gain nothing. Let them think about your so-called inability to get patients. Rely upon your hard work and pay full attention to professional ethics and you will see that you gain money in due course of time. If you do not work hard and are worried about what others think about you, you will end up feeling guilty even when you have earned money by sheer luck. If you are overflowing with money, you will have fear of losing it. The core 'mantra' to earn money and respect money is to work hard and leave every thing to luck. Luck will not fail you if you, work hard.

LUST FOR COMPETITION : BEST FRIEND

Coming to competition, it must be understood that those in competition with you in the market also faced the same thing when they entered the field. Competition has always existed in every market and still people are earning. Competition is major phenomenon and one has to struggle for recognition in the market. Now think deeply about this term competition. You will find that competition is nothing but lack of something. May be it is lack of money, lack of patients, lack of space to work and lack of good prime location for clinic. If it is within your resources to remove the 'lacks', the competition is over but it is not possible to do so. The competition remains. Understanding this, one can feel that everything is in abundance in the market. You lack something and it is you to make lack into abundance by use of little inguinity. You should stand out from others. For example, a new clinic can have less of consultation fee, medicines at the daily rates instead of weeks supply, free consultation to the poor, declaring the clinic a speciality for children or women diseases etc. You can very well write on the clinic display board 'special care and cure for the old'. There is no speciality required for such type of inscriptions. This is one example. Use your genuine and innovative ideas of getting attention from the public.

Three most important values for a new entrant in profession of Homoeopathy

- Judge what you need.
- Decide how to fulfill the need?
- Make it happen.

Bibliography

Organon of medicine	S.Hahnemann
Repertory of Homoeopathic Materia Medica	J. T. Kent
Boenninghausen's Therapeutic Pocket Book	H. A. Roberts and Annie C. Wilson
Comparative Materia Medica and Therapeutics	N. C. Ghosh
Homoeopathic Materia Medica and Repertory	W. Boerick
Keynotes of Leading Remedies	H.C.Allen
Prescriber	John H. Clarke
Materia Medica	C. Hering
Select Your Remedy	R.B.Bishamber Das
Bedside Prescriber	J. N. Singhal
The Principle and Art of Cure by Homoeopathy	H. A. Roberts
Practice of Medicine	F. W. Price
Highlights of Homoeopathic Practicing	T. P. Chatterjee
Human Anatomy and Physiology	V. Tatarinov
Essentials of Homoeopathic Materia Medica and Pharmacy	W. A. Dewey
Homoeopathic Prescriber	K. C. Bhanja
Hom. Family practice	Bhattacharya
Domestic physician	Constantine Hering
Practioner's guide to Gall bladder stones and Kidney stones	Shiv Dua
Oral Diseases	Shiv Dua
Neck pain, Cervical Spondylosis	Shiv Dua
Know and solve your Thyroid Problems	Shiv Dua

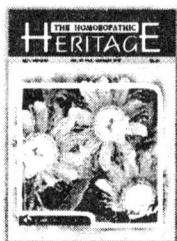

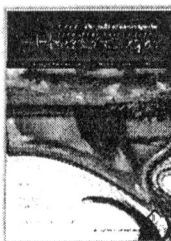

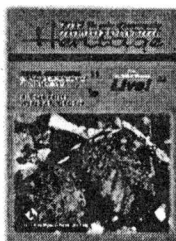